CODES OF LONGEVITY

Be Ageless - Live Limitless

Learn from 20+ of Today's Leading Health Experts How to Unlock Your Potential to Look, Feel and Live Life Optimized to 120 and Beyond!

DR. MELISSA GRILL-PETERSEN

CODES OF LONGEVITY

Transcendent Publishing
PO Box 66202
St. Pete Beach, FL 33736
www.TranscendentPublishing.com

Paperback ISBN: 978-1-7353738-5-0
eBook ISBN: 978-1-7353738-6-7

Disclaimer: This book is not intended to diagnose, treat, cure, or prevent any disease and is not intended to be the medical advice of a physician. You should, before you act or use any of this information, consider the appropriateness of this information having regard to your own personal situation and needs. You are responsible for consulting a suitable medical professional before using any of the information or materials contained in this book or accessed through any electronic means before trying any treatment or taking any course of action that may directly or indirectly affect your health or wellbeing.

For the complete list of references for this book, visit: www.codesoflongevity.com

Printed in the United States of America

To my husband Jim, thank you for all of your love, allowing me to be me, while supporting my vision and our family every day. I love you.

For my son Topher, you inspire and remind me every day of the pure potential that life holds. May you always share your light and remember you are limitless!

For my tribe and co-authors, thank you for adding your genius to this narrative as together we remind the world and one another how to express our potential to be the change we wish to see.

CONTENTS

FOREWORD

Welcome to the tipping point.

The moment in time where we as a collective have begun to contemplate the potential for a life where we have a choice. Rapid advancement of scientific knowledge along with accelerating technologies have extended the horizon of possibilities for experiences previously thought to be unobtainable. We ride the front edge of a wave of unprecedented expansion that will drive innovations which propel an intentional evolution of the human species. This evolution will result in an increase not only in lifespan but in healthspan, a shift from decaying and dying to age reversal and purposeful thriving. A leap from the concept of wellbeing to a state of MORE Being.

Get ready to take a deep dive into this exciting journey of new, enhanced possibilities for extending lifespan and healthspan. Dr. Melissa has assembled a group of experts featured within the upcoming pages that are leaders in the health optimization and precision longevity industry. Together they share their individual expertise as a part of a larger system or body of knowledge revealing how each piece of the longevity puzzle fits together for a new expression of health and thriving.

I have personally been immersed in the deep and often cloudy waters of the age rejuvenation arena since early 2005. Most of us involved in this pursuit in the early days were considered a bit out there and indeed perhaps even a little crazy, yet as with all true visionaries we were not deterred as we knew the possibilities, and this was enough to keep us vectored toward the future state. I remember speaking at a conference in 2014 where I presented the coming landscape of age reversal; I laid out the primary nine hallmarks of aging that would need to be addressed to move the marker on our potential to get there.

Unfortunately, the tools we needed were not yet available. I predicted that we would more than likely see the reality of the first valid interventions within the next five years. I am grateful to say that we now have validated these early strategies.

These nine hallmarks were first published by *Lopez-Otin et al* in the publication **CELL** in Nov. 2013 titled ***The Hallmarks of Aging***. They include genomic instability, telomere shortening, epigenetic alterations, loss of proteostasis, dysregulated nutrient sensing, mitochondrial dysfunction, cell senescence, stem cell loss, and altered intercellular communication. These discoveries provide us with an opportunity to create interventions which mitigate the ravages of ageing and importantly, provide the ability to rejuvenate the aging system to a place of youthful longevity.

From Possibility to Reality

In September of 2019, Gregory Fahy and Steven Horvath published a small study in *Aging Cell* entitled "Reversal of epigenetic aging and immunosenescence trends in humans." In their paper, they reported on nine individuals who underwent a year of a simple therapy of growth hormone injections, DHEA, metformin, Vitamin D3, and zinc. I purposefully use the word simple here because this is a common therapeutic approach used by many "anti-aging" clinics and there are programs utilizing much more advanced interventions with subsequent stunning success. This published clinical trial in particular measured aging according to epigenetic profiles developed by Dr. Horvath along with assessment of the youthfulness of the immune system.

> *Epigenetic age is a tool to assess biologic age as opposed to chrono-*
> *logic age. Biologic age measures methylation (modifications to*
> *your DNA that can change its expression) and is based on years*
> *of statistical research. These methylation "marks" tend to ac-*
> *cumulate as we age and correlate with a biologic age, risk of*
> *chronic disease, and how many years you have left.*

The study, called the TRIIM (Thymus Regeneration, Immuno-
restoration, and Insulin Mitigation) trial ran from 2015-2017 and the
results were impressive. The results showed that there was
epigenetic age reversal of 2.5 years! This was an important study
because prior to this point most researchers felt that epigenetic
aging was a one direction process, and this opened the possibility
that age *REVERSAL* was actually a potential.

What is Aging?

One of the issues currently under debate in the scientific community is the question of what is aging? It is not a difficult question
to answer as we observe this process every day from a biological
standpoint, yet "aging" is a complex phenomenon to describe. Is
aging an actual process or is it a constellation of diverse isolated
processes that we have mentally grouped together? The debate
now posits that even if we identify all of these processes, will we be
able to have a real impact that will prolong lifespan and more
importantly extend health-span? Some researchers believe that
there is an evolutionarily selected programming in our DNA that
instructs the system to age. It seems that the more we discover, the
more questions we find which require answers.

Does this mean that extended healthy longevity is out of our reach?
A dream in what might be considered a fairytale. No, I do not
believe that it is.

What I do believe is that this will require a new approach to health
and biology, one that will require doctors and researchers to

dispense with the current model of looking at life through a linear lens and adopt instead a paradigm of seeing the human system for the complex adaptive system it is. Linear biology is based on implicit and explicit concepts, assumptions, and beliefs. In our current medical model, the human system is based on reductionist and deterministic processes, yet this is not how the human system works.

What I mean by this is that the human system has been treated as though it responds in a linear fashion – input A = output B, if you double A then it will double the output B. Complex adaptive systems do not work this way. A complex adaptive system is one that is made up of multiple local agents interacting with one another through local feedback systems which have unpredictable net outcomes across and within the whole system. When we begin to view the human system through this complex lens, we can then design and test interventions with a true understanding of complex biologic systems such as "aging." It also possesses emergent properties, meaning that with repeated exposure to environmental conditions, the system will adapt in order to function better and so the same input will then create a different, or emergent, property that changes the response.

How Far Away Are We?

This is a common question I hear often when I speak about age rejuvenation. The encouraging answer I give, is that we are getting closer. We have seen massive amounts of private investment into companies in this space over the past several years and it is increasing every year. We are currently experiencing a shift in the worldview around age reversal and extended health-span. This is an important phenomenon because until the pervasive opinion on the possibility of age reversal shifts toward "yes, it might be possible," then progress will remain slow. Along with this we are witnessing exponential growth in scientific knowledge and technologies which will further speed up the process.

Will there be a pill or a treatment that will miraculously pull off a Benjamin Buttons type of response? No, certainly not. What we are more likely to see is gradual development of interventions that will rejuvenate individual body systems back a few years and keep us alive and healthy long enough for the next intervention to come along. This will be a bit like two steps forward and three steps back (as in three years younger).

What is Available for Us Now?

The answer here is, it depends. What I mean by this is that there are many interventions available now, but we do not have the longitudinal studies to inform on their effectiveness or long-term safety. That said, there are many of us who are not willing to wait for these longitudinal studies because, let's be real, most of us will be dead before the results of the long-term studies are well documented. This is why we are seeing a surge of biohackers, self-experimenters, and first adopters taking the process into their own hands. I prefer to refer to this most adventurous community as the n of 1's, essentially they use sense-making, professional guidance, and feedback through testing and measurements to understand how these interventions impact their system. There are a few clinicians that support these sovereign individuals in their ventures and several companies creating offshore sites where they can work with these individuals outside of governmental restrictions. We have been working with a lot of leading-edge interventions in our clinic that still align with regulations and yet few people know of the availability.

Whether you are the more adventurous type or slightly reserved, there are still plenty of interventions available now. The first and foremost intervention available to everyone is lifestyle. This is the foundation from which all interventions will build from and yet it is one that few are willing to entertain perhaps because they may be confused about what a healthy lifestyle plan encompasses.

This book offers a beginning point on your precision longevity path that can be personalized for you. The book's experienced authors understand complexity thinking and how it informs health. Most have trained in advanced genetic and epigenetic strategies and tactics at the Aperion Academy and have a solid grasp of helping people to identify a personalized plan that aligns with their goals and motivation to optimize and enhance their human system.

What you will discover more about in the upcoming pages are the same processes we utilize with our clients to achieve age rejuvenation and maintain youthful longevity:

- **Lifestyle** – Sleep optimization practices, precision nutrition plans customized to an individual's genetics and goals, specific exercise protocols that have shown clinical evidence to boost longevity, a strategic environmental design map, and work with optimizing the autonomic and central nervous system to create an anti-fragile state of stress response and resilience.

- **Hormone optimization** - Find a physician that understands the complexity of the body's hormonal symphony and the benefits of having youthful levels.

- **Senolytics** - Senolytics are the new power packed, heavy hitters of longevity and rejuvenation. These compounds address one of the major common pathways of age reversal as they target nearly all of the nine hallmarks of aging. Each senolytic has different cell type targets and must be used strategically and in an intermittent fashion. There are several of these available by prescription but there are also some very powerful supplements that have a proven ability to reduce the numbers of these cells.

- **Immunity** - Immune cells and thymic gland function are greatly impacted in the aging human system. Rejuvenation of this system is addressed via multiple pathways. Mammalian target of rapamycin, (mTOR) activity is essential for growth and development, it tends not to downregulate once we are done maturing, this creates potential detrimental effects. Turning down this activity has been shown to decrease cancer incidence, improve cardiac function, improve general health, and increase lifespan. The thymus gland is a significant source of our cellular immunity and it tends to stop working completely by our early 30's. Human trials have shown that specific interventions can turn this back on again, as seen in the TRIIM trial, resulting in boosting the immune system. Again, there are prescriptions for this as well as over the counter supplements.

- **DNA Repair** - In the aging human the surveillance and maintenance systems involved in DNA repair become less and less efficient. We provide several interventions that support and upregulate this process. Decreasing levels of NAD+ has been a focal point of this loss of efficiency and despite a host of proclaimed interventions to boost this system, few have actually proven therapeutic. We have been able to remove the hype and focus on interventions that truly create better NAD+ response.

You will learn many more details in this book from experts in their particular subject but each of these authors also understands that a whole system approach is necessary in order to make a real impact. This is an exciting subject, one that is constantly improving and advancing daily. The material in this book is well established at this point and is a great starting point for anyone on this journey.

I invite you to integrate the information in this book, to contemplate what makes sense to you and to take action on those things that resonate. I encourage you to join me in the quest to enhance the human experience and intentionally evolve our species as we move from a state of limited separation consciousness to one of limitless unity consciousness. The future is ours to design and script, let's accept the reins and guide it purposefully. Our very thriving depends on it.

Yours in Limitless Expression!
Daniel Stickler, MD
Co-Founder of Apeiron Zoh

Dr. Daniel Stickler *is the Co-Founder and Chief Medical Officer of The Apeiron Center for Human Potential and Chief Science Officer for Apeiron Academy. He is the visionary pioneer behind systems-based precision lifestyle medicine, a new paradigm that redefines medicine from the old symptoms-based disease model to one of limitless peak performance in all aspects of life.*

A physician to high-performing executives and entrepreneurs who want to upgrade their current state, he's also an author, speaker, blogger and podcaster. He is the Medical Director for the Neurohacker Collective, a Google consultant for wearable technology, epigenetics, and AI in healthcare and a guest lecturer at Stanford University on Epigenetics in Clinical Practice.

www.ApeironZoh.com

INTRODUCTION

Welcome to the new era of ageless living. I'm excited to share the experts, science and insights brought together in this book to tell a new story of what is possible in living a long and thriving life. Consider this book your field guide of sorts designed to reveal how to unlock your codes of longevity so you can look, feel and live your life optimized at any age.

A few years ago, I got to thinking about the images and messages the media floods our screens with every day. As if reading my mind, up pops a commercial showing a mom in pain struggling to make it through her day. The next scene shows her happy and pain-free thanks to the medication followed by the warning of the many side effects. My son was watching this with me and asked, "Why would anyone want to take that? Listen to all of the ways it can be bad for you; how is that possibly good?"

It was in the next breath I said to him, what do you imagine it would be like if every day instead of commercials telling us what's wrong with us, telling us we need something to "fix us," we were told what's right? What if we were shown images of thriving individuals tapping into their limitless potential? How differently might we all be walking around living our lives and expressing vitality?

The brain seeks proof to validate what is possible. The 4-minute mile was said to be impossible until it wasn't. As soon as Roger Bannister broke that barrier, within two months his competitors began doing the same. What was believed to be impossible became possible.

We are sitting at that same breakthrough point where what it means to be human at any age is being redefined. The ability to do more than survive as we move through life is causing people worldwide to seek new ways to thrive. The promise to do this easily to 120 and beyond is now the new 4-minute mile ready to be achieved.

For more than 20 years as a doctor, author, speaker and leader in the wellness space, I have known with 100% certainty of the infinite potential within each person to heal, flourish and optimize any aspect of their health or life. I have never seen anyone as broken, limited or lacking but rather a diamond ready to shine. It's been in seeing each person's wholeness, understanding their potential and working through a systems-based approach that has allowed me to support them to break through the limitations they had placed on themselves into new expressions of thriving.

It is this same knowing that I bring to you through this book. This is my mission, to share with you what IS possible in hopes that you will gain insights to be inspired, informed and ignited in new ways to express your highest outcomes and live your best life. Regardless of what you have thought or been told, if you desire more, you are in the right place. If you sense that more is possible, that you can live a life of energy, vitality, meaning, connection and joy, you're right, you can. If you believe that age is just a number, that 50 is the new 30, and 100 is the new 70, you are among like minds. If you sense that aging is optional and you want a clear understanding of how to discern the breakthrough science and solutions for a personalized precision longevity plan so you can be ageless and live limitless, then keep reading.

While exciting breakthroughs are being reported daily in the longevity space, much confusion still exists.

Is it good genes, stem cells, nutrition, biohacks, a top dermatologist or surgeon, hormones, serums, or some fountain of youth known only to a few? What about the countless stories of people who smoke and drink and live to be a hundred – what are their secrets? On the other hand, what goes wrong when someone who is vegan and runs ten miles a day does not make it to their thirty-fifth birthday?

That's where this book comes in. In the pages that follow you will meet me and my co-authors who are trailblazing healthcare practitioners and thought leaders constantly shining a light into the new discoveries, beyond the preconceived notions around aging. Together we will explore what really IS possible and how we can each access and apply the new science, along with ancient wisdom and traditions, to live a longer life than we ever thought possible and, just as importantly, live it well.

You will see that aging is not a disease, but a process that with the right tools you can stop, slow down and even reverse. More importantly, you will understand the choices available to you right now to support your body, mind and spirit to increase your lifespan and healthspan far beyond the current norms.

Cracking the longevity code requires a systems approach, one based on the reality that you are one whole body, interacting with the world around you. You are not one pathway, one cell, one process, but a bio-dynamic human organism that is constantly being informed through trillions of signals each and every moment of each and every day.

The signals from the outerworld – your daily environment, thoughts, habits, actions and beliefs – transfer key information to the innerworld of your body. Your body, which is more than one organ or system, is a whole system working together for your greatest expression of health and vitality. We will take a deeper look into three keys:

- **Lifespan** is the span of time or number of years you will live. While lifespan in general is increasing around the globe, we are not gaining quality of life. This has caused researchers to ask why. This led to the discovery of the nine hallmarks of aging that define how and why we age from a physiological standpoint. Think of these as the biological markers that influence the rate of aging in the body. Complete with an easy-to-understand explanation of the specific components that can affect the length of our lives, we will explore how to influence lifespan for more years and greater health through genetics and stem cells to sirtuins, clocks, nutrients and more.

- **Healthspan** is the quality of our health over the years. Influenced heavily through lifestyle and environment, you will discover the most significant levers that can be adjusted to slow down or reverse the aging process to feel great, and have the energy, strength and vitality to enjoy life, for as long as we live.

- **Wellspan** is a new concept we are adding to this systems-based approach to enhancing longevity. Just looking at cellular biology, we understand that bio hacks and lifestyle alone do not necessarily add up to a long and vital life. As found in any "bluezone," wellbeing is a central component to living long and living well. This "secret sauce" encompasses things like connection and a sense of purpose, as well as social, economic and emotional support, all of which enhance the quality of one's life and plays a vital role in designing your optimal longevity blueprint.

These sections reveal the essential codes to inform and activate your potential embedded in your DNA to be ageless. Consider each an interlocking piece and part that add up to make the whole picture of what creates longevity. Historically, each "code" has been treated as an individual input missing the understanding of how it informs the system overall. When you recognize each, you can begin to connect them together for exponential impact, to slow down and reverse age to look and feel your best ongoing.

AGELESSNESS

The timeless in you is aware of life's timelessness.
It knows that yesterday is but today's memory
And tomorrow is today's dream.

-Khalil Gibran

CHAPTER ONE

Unlock Your Code
Be Ageless - Live Limitless

Dr. Melissa Grill-Petersen

If you knew you had all of the resources you needed to live your life fully, meeting your goals and aspirations, how long and how well would you want to live?

Once you've achieved those goals, would you want to end there? What if there could be even more to your story?

The power of story is set in motion, influencing our conscious and unconscious mind from the moment of conception. Informed through the DNA, brought to life by our "cultural editors." Parents, teachers, media, our heritage, religion and more are all telling us every day who we are and what is possible, yet what if their story is not fully yours?

To unlock your codes of longevity begins within the mind. This is where you hold your personal values, desires and beliefs of what is possible for you. Understanding what you deeply desire and why is the first place in gaining clarity around your own inner narrative. Your personal story that will act as your guidance system revealing what does or does not align with the very outcomes you seek.

Right now, you may have no idea how long you want to live, you just know that today, in this moment, you want to be the best expression of yourself. That is the perfect place to begin…

Find Your Longevity Potential

Let's prime your longevity mind to find a realistic framework of what IS possible for you. This is called the longevity potential formula inspired by Dr. Eric Plasker of the 100-year lifestyle.

1. Determine the age of your oldest living relative. This could be a great grandparent, parent, aunt, uncle etc.

2. Subtract your current age today from the age of the oldest living relative.

3. The difference is the minimum amount of years you will likely live.

EX: My great grandmother lived to 95 – my current age of 49 = 55

Now that you have a starting point of how long you can easily live (this is before all of the age reversing strategies that add more years to the clock for you), the real question is, *HOW do you want to be living?*

Do you desire to be vital, joyful, creative, connected, energized, clear, loved and loving, healthy, playful and strong? Do you seek new adventures, new discoveries, and new ways of contributing to and impacting the world?

Your wants, vision, desires and beliefs are all available to you, desiring you as you them.

Yet, desire alone isn't always enough, especially when it conflicts with our inner stories told to us over a lifetime by others. If you have ever both wanted something deeply yet felt resistance to it at the same moment, that's inner opposition revealing itself between your conscious and unconscious mind. A tug between what you want and what others want for you.

You know you've hit a roadblock when you feel even the slightest bit of resistance. You can be going through your day feeling great and then a moment occurs when you feel it – you are triggered, taken out of your flow. These are unconscious cues of our inner programming – the ideas, philosophies, understandings, systems, definitions of how life is to be and how we are to be within it – that were made up by others and passed down, generation to generation, through our cultural editors.

I felt this as I began writing this book. I know both through science and my own beliefs that we can live to 120 and beyond in a thriving state. My personal story of what is possible for myself and humanity is clear and strong yet, in the very next moment, doubt entered my mind, creating roadblocks of uncertainty.

While I personally want to create a long, fully vibrant life, I am reminded of my mother who was diagnosed with cancer at age fifty-two and made her transition just after her fifty-fourth birthday. Her story ended very differently from the one I desire to experience for myself.

Yes, I consciously know that her journey is not mine. I also fully understand that I don't have to fear the curse of "genetics." Thanks to the science of epigenetics, we know that our genes do not dictate our destiny.

Think of the genetic code like a recipe of potential. Each letter of your code, ingredients, yet alone the ingredients do not make the meal. It is the amount of each, the ways they are combined, and how long they are cooked that determine the end result. In other words, while I may have similar genetic ingredients as my mother, it is my perception, response and interaction to my daily environment, along with lifestyle that will be the main influence on how my genes will express.

Although I live my life much differently from the way she did and I have all of the knowledge that should bring me comfort, I am still haunted by her fate.

If left unresolved, this could become a limitation I place on my own potential.

If left unexplored, I may ask myself big questions, set grandiose visions and plans, and still find myself living small. Living someone else's story instead of experiencing my own.

This is where my beliefs didn't line up consciously and unconsciously. My fear of my mother's fate becoming my own was overriding my conscious desires.

So how is it done? How can the limiting stories or beliefs that seem to be lodged in our unconscious brain from another time or space be transformed? How can we identify these stories, patterns, or beliefs that no longer serve us and shift them into new possibilities, understandings, and truths that support our highest expression?

Access Your Ageless Mind

In comes the mind hacks – questions that can reveal boundaries, highlight possibility and potential, to uncover the answers that can and will immediately align you with your now truth. As new understandings emerge, new definitions, beliefs and values can be created to fully serve the you of now, rather than the you of twenty years ago.

I wear many titles yet at my core, I'm a transformational coach, who for more than twenty years has helped thousands – and myself – upgrade their brains, bodies, businesses and lives. Luckily, I also have incredible coaches around me, as we all need another to hold up a mirror through which we can have our individual a-ha moments. In fact, just last week I had an unexpected longevity breakthrough thanks to my friend and high-performance coach, Meg Foley.

As I was interviewing her, she decided to make me her subject to show a mind hack session in real time. Since we were talking about creating an ageless mind, she suggested I identify the word that I associated with living a long life. I immediately said "aging" and thought this was strange as it seems the exact opposite of living a long life.

Meg then prompted me to ask myself several times over to *fully explore and consider what the word "aging" means to me.*

My answers began to flood in as I said it means slowing down, becoming frail, low energy, shrinking, becoming decrepit. We noticed that as I was saying these words, my body was visibly taking on showing the posture of aging!

Next she asked me to consider, *What if everything I think I know about "aging" is all wrong?* This was fascinating, for when I asked myself that question my mind immediately expanded. I started saying, "What if aging really isn't frailty at all, but freedom? What if, instead of slowing down it means adventure?" And on I went, exploring the newfound answers.

Then she asked, "Why is it important for you to want to live a long life?" to which I immediately replied, "I love my life and family, and for me, longevity is really about being able to spend as much time with them, and doing what I love, for as long as possible. This fills me up, brings me joy and is everything to me."

What we uncovered is that my core is *connection*. Living a long life is about enjoying connection with all that I love.

Meg then asked me if my current definition of aging will support me in fully enjoying this level of connection that means so much to me too, which of course I answered no.

That is the moment I was able to consciously acknowledge that my original understanding no longer serves me, and that what really matters to me is to live a long thriving life of love and connection. As a result, my boundaries were *immediately expanded*. My brain took a quantum leap into a new, consciously aligned state of longevity and thriving – one that will manifest as daily opportunities to experience and express my best health and self in order to connect with everyone and everything I love for as long as possible.

In this same moment, I realized, my mother's definitions of how she saw her path, longevity and life were much different than mine. The limitation of fear dissipated, regardless of my lifespan, I now have total certainty of what it means to me.

For my mother, what she saw for herself was a life of limitation. She didn't know how to trust her body; she was constantly living with the reminder of discomfort and dysfunction. That was too painful for her to want to stick around, she couldn't see more as possible. For me, I see a life of pure potential, infinite moments of connection, adventure and so much yet to come that I am excited and joyful of what my journey will bring.

While this does not guarantee me any certain lifespan, what I now have is a wholeness in my aligned connection between my desire and definitions. Through answering a few questions, I updated the stories that I had been told or told myself.

Set Your Longevity Life Vision

You, right now, have the power to re-write or newly design your story. Let it express your highest outcomes for what you want, desire and deserve in creating and living your longevity life.

I invite you to use this framework to now consider and gain clarity around your desires and definitions when it comes to optimal health, aging and longevity.

Are these definitions aligned with the life you truly want to live?

Now is the time to get curious. Now is the time to design the ideal length and quality of your life. Think of it as your guiding light, your map to keep you headed in the direction of where you most desire to go during your life adventure.

- **Step One: Set Your Vision.** What does longevity look like and mean to you, in terms of your own life? Really dial into what you will be doing, how you will be feeling, who you will be with, what resources you have, and the highest expression you desire to live.

- **Step Two: Identify Your Roadblocks.** What, if any, feelings, emotions or beliefs come up as a potential doubt or in contrast to your vision? Is it safe for you to live the life you desire? Are you worthy of experiencing what you want?

- **Step Three: Find Your Word.** Give your roadblock a word (for me it was aging). Ask yourself, "What does the word _____ mean to me?" then write down everything that comes to you. What are the associations you make to that word, feeling or state of being?

- **Step Four: Find Your Why.** Why don't you want to experience your roadblocks, and why DO you want to experience your vision of a long life? Is there a natural theme that shows up for you? For me it was a thriving life of connection. Why is living your long life to the fullest important to you?

- **Step Five: Flip Reality.** Ask yourself, "What if everything I thought I knew about _____ (insert your word) is wrong?"

- **Step Six: What Do You Notice Now?** What definitions or boundaries, if any, have shifted for you during this exercise? How has your mindset expanded? What new understandings do you now have regarding what is possible for you in experiencing a long healthy life?

Let this new awareness of what you desire guide you as you read the rest of this book. You will find it reveals the many ways in which you can create your personalized path to a long, abundant and thriving life.

Ageless Mind Challenge

Do you want to experience the power of your ageless mind in action? Get ready to look and feel more youthful, vital and strong without any lotions, potions or pills in as little as one week when you take the seven-day age reversal challenge. Find out more at www.TheCodesofLongevity.com.

CHAPTER TWO

The End of Aging

Dr. Melissa Grill-Petersen

Welcome to the forefront of life extension. Today, science is revealing the processes responsible for why the body ages and why we don't have to.

In the previous chapter we explored your definition of longevity and your ideal vision of a long and happy life; we also identified possible roadblocks you may have unintentionally placed in your way. I now invite you to imagine that every moment of this vision has been captured in a wide-angle camera lens, providing the BIG macro picture of your life. If you were to zoom in frame by frame, you would be able to see each piece of that picture in great detail.

It is by zooming in and out that we can gain an understanding of how it is possible to slow down, stop and even reverse the aging process. As we do so, going from the expansive image of our highest vision and desired expression of our life ahead, down to the cellular level in the body, and back out again, we see how each action, interaction and moment in the outworld affects the whole of us, positively or negatively. In other words, the process of zooming in and out helps us make sense of how lifespan, healthspan and wellspan all connect, stack and layer upon one another to create our expression of optimized health.

Once you have this understanding of these moving parts, you can determine what immediate, short- and long-term opportunities exist for you to take to turn back your clock and gain years of quality life. This phenomenon is called the *longevity escape velocity*, by which science is discovering how to extend life by more than a year for every year you are alive. There are several incredible advancements on the horizon that will help them do this, a key example of which is the development of 3-D printed organs, which are coming to market as early as 2023. Genetic therapies also bring many potential solutions with them; in fact, researchers estimate they can eradicate over 32,000 diseases with CRISPR, a tool through which they can actually edit DNA and genetic expression. These, along with solutions designed to enhance cellular health and function, tell us that disease and organ failure can become a thing of the past, and the era of age reversal is here to stay.

While the very near future holds these and other exciting possibilities, there is still a missing piece to the longevity puzzle. This is where the analogy of zooming in and out comes into play. Currently, most scientists, researchers, inventors and practitioners are "zoomed in," meaning they approach the new breakthroughs in longevity only through their lens of their own specialty, without "zooming out" to see how these components affect the whole. To use another analogy, they are focused on the pebble dropped into the pond, rather than the ripple effect that pebble creates across the entire body of water.

For example, when we zoom into the inner world of the body, we can answer the foundational question: What causes the body to age? Then, to understand a systems view, we move back out, adjusting our lens to see more of the picture, including our thoughts, habits, and interactions with our daily environment (the outer world). We can then begin to see how the way one perceives, interacts and experiences the outworld informs the key biological processes that will either speed up, slow down or reverse the aging process within the body. It is this knowledge that gives us power over ourselves, and direct access to the codes that will support us in designing lives that extend years, even decades, past the current norms.

The coming chapters will seek to fill this gap by sharing a systems-based approach that demystifies and simplifies how and where lifespan, healthspan and wellspan intersect, like those ripples in the water, to create an enhanced expression of a thriving life. First, though, we'll begin with some foundational information that will give you a greater understanding of each of these areas.

What Causes the Body to Age?

In an interview we did together, Aubry De Grey provided a simple explanation of aging as the buildup of metabolic damage in the body that, over time, leads to pathology. It is through the targeting of metabolic processes, therefore, that we have the potential to slow down and reverse aging.

Lifespan, is the current understanding of how long we can chronologically live, and is thought to be driven by certain "hallmarks of aging." First published by *Lopez-Otin et al* in the publication **CELL** in Nov. 2013 titled *The Hallmarks of Aging*, they are also, for our purposes here, the codes to understanding the biological processes in the body that impact longevity.

The first three are considered "primary," from which each additional hallmark is affected. This top-down or bottom-up approach begs the question: What are the triggers that set this cascade in motion? You will notice as you read through these that they are all impacted by lifestyle and environment (healthspan factors), thus setting the stage for how the outer world is in fact impacting the expression of health, or aging, in the inner world.

1. **Genomic Instability**: Your genes house the code of YOU. Life and the daily exposures to it over time can create less stability that leads to breakdown and damage.

    According to the book, understanding genetics, *cells are the fundamental structural and functional units of every known living organism. Instructions needed to direct activities are contained within a DNA (deoxyribonucleic acid) sequence. DNA from all organisms is made up of the same chemical units (bases) called adenine, thymine, guanine, and cytosine, abbreviated as A, T, G, and C. In complementary DNA strands, A matches with T, and C with G, to form base pairs.*

Genes are specific sequences of bases that encode instructions for how to make proteins. Each gene has a unique DNA sequence. Although each cell contains a full complement of DNA, cells use genes selectively. For example, the genes active in a liver cell differ from the genes active in a brain cell because each cell performs different functions and, therefore, requires different proteins. Different genes can also be activated during development or in response to environmental stimuli such as an infection or stress. It is the inputs, stimuli or signals from the environment that inform the DNA how to express, this is the science of epigenetics (to be further discussed throughout this book).

It is the very exposure to our daily world that is the first and main contributor to the aging process. While the body is designed to correct the damage to the DNA, it is reported that an average individual experiences hundreds of thousands of breaks in the DNA each day. Think of this like your car breaking down and requiring maintenance. While DNA breaks are part of the "normal wear and tear" in the body, modern living has added in new stressors that are increasing the rate and degree to which repair is needed. The more this occurs, the greater the need for proper resources within the body to correct the damage. Too often, we are not giving our body enough of what it needs to offset the damage and inflammation creating an inability to keep up and instability sets in. This increased need for repair also increases the rate of mistakes during repair, causing damage that impacts the entire system. Some of these stressors are brought on by our environment, such as exposure to toxins, pollutants, UV radiation, reactive oxygen species (think of these like rust in the cells), carcinogens and tobacco.

If your very code isn't able to properly repair, you aren't thriving. In fact, you accelerate the chance for disease through the accumulation of mutated cells that are rendered "dysfunctional." At this point, the mutated cells *should* die through a built-in safety mechanism of self-suicide called apoptosis; however, many cells avoid this fate and slip into another stage known as cellular scenescence.

The senescent cells, also referred to as "zombie cells," no longer divide or support the tissue they are a part of while emitting chemical signals that can turn other cells in the area to a senescent state. In later chapters, my co-authors will share the ways in which to reduce your exposure to these triggers and support the clearing of senescent cells, as well as how to enhance cellular health through proper sirtuin activation, NAD and mitochondrial efficiency for improved function over time.

2. **Telomere Attrition** - Telomeres are the protective caps on the ends of our chromosomes. They ensure proper DNA replication and act as a clock monitoring the lifespan through how many times each chromosome can replicate. The greatest challenge posed by telomere attrition is that, over time, healthy cells diminish, leading to poor system function and the accumulation of senescent cells, which in turn results in chronic inflammation and damage to the surrounding tissue. Lifestyle factors such as increased weight, tobacco use, alcohol consumption, pollution, emotional and environmental stressors are some of the biggest drivers to this type of breakdown. One of the best ways to clear senescent cells and mitigate this "metaflammation" is

through time-restricted eating and intermittent fasting, which is discussed in upcoming chapters.

3. **Epigenetic Alterations**. Epigenetics are the signals from "above the gene" that cue genetic expression. It's important to understand that all of the different types of cells in your body, from liver and muscle cells to immune, glial cells and more, ALL have the exact same genetic code. The DNA is the same for every single one of the trillions of cells in our body. What determines how those cells express in their individual form is the epigenome. Think of the DNA as the hardware of the computer and the epigenome as the software, or the DNA as the ingredients and the epigenome as the recipe that informs how those ingredients are mixed to make a specific meal.

   The epigenome is the environment around the cell that "informs" or signals the DNA. Influencers on this environment include both your physical environment – the world around you – and how you are perceiving and interacting within that world, which as mentioned previously informs and affects the inner environment of the body.

   Alterations such as mutation, RNA degradation, methylation and histone modification can all "silence" the gene, in essence turning it off and impairing normal function.

   Factors such as diet, obesity, physical activity, tobacco use/ smoking, alcohol consumption, environmental pollutants, psychological stress, and working night shifts modify epigenetic patterns leading to alterations in the function of the DNA.

This is the tipping point, where the genetic impact (informed and influenced from lifestyle and environment) of the first three hallmarks now continues in a downstream effect in the body to influence the additional markers of aging.

4. **Loss of Proteostasis.** Proteostasis is a homeostatic state that ensures proper folding and function of protein cells within the body. Proteins do much more than build muscle; they also regulate almost every function in the body either directly or indirectly. They are made up of smaller amino acids, the sequence of which depends upon the structure and function of the protein and the exact role it will carry out in the body. Aging impairs this process and can cause unfolded, misfolded or aggregate proteins that can lead to pathology such as Alzheimer's. Genetic and epigenetic alterations, changes in pH, environmental stressors, the accumulation of advanced glycation end products (AGEs) and oxidation (rust in the cells) can initiate a loss of proteostasis. This is a key point where breakdown in communication can occur within the expression of health in the body.

5. **Deregulated Nutrient Sensing.** This results from a breakdown of proper function in the four primary longevity nutrient-sensing pathways: IIS (insulin and IGF-1) and mTOR (anabolic pathways), along with AMPK and sirtuins (the catabolic pathways). Think of high mTOR and IIS activity like the phrase "Live fast, die young," because too much activity is good for growth but bad for lifespan. However, too little mTOR activity is not beneficial either, as studies have shown it can disrupt healing and insulin sensitivity. This can occur from too much of certain nutrients and/or stressors to the system that disturb the balance, for example by increasing IIS and mTOR or decreasing AMPK and sirtuin activation.

AMPK ensures proper cellular energy and autophagy – or adequate ATP production and the removal of senescent cells, respectively. If dysregulated, metaflammation increases intra- and extracellularly and overall energy production, healing and repair all decline.

Sirtuins, which are discussed at length in later chapters, play a key role in regulating cellular homeostasis. Cells *are the fundamental structural and functional units of every known living organism.* Homeostasis involves keeping the cell in balance and working optimally. Sirtuins are key drivers in cellular health, however, they can only function in the presence of NAD+, nicotinamide adenine dinucleotide, a coenzyme found in all living cells. When the body is unable to properly recognize, utilize or process essential nutrients required for the system to express health, and support the production of NAD+ within the cell, metabolic chaos ensues.

6. **Mitochondrial Dysfunction.** The mitochondria are known as the powerhouse of your cells. They act like miniature factories, converting the food we eat into usable energy, adenosine triphosphate (ATP). This process creates reactive oxygen species (ROS) known as free-radicals or oxidative stress, which play a key role in cellular health but over time and with increased accumulation are associated with in-flammaging, immune suppression, frailty, senescent cells, and mutations that can cause cancers. This hallmark, which is brought on by environmental and lifestyle factors, can be addressed by activating the AMPK and Sirtuin pathways and increasing NAD+ to support mitochondrial function, as well as the removal of toxins, pathogens or metaflammation that impact the delivery of nutrients into the cell.

7. **Cellular Senescence**: As a person ages, there is an increase in senescent or "zombie cells" described above. It is therefore essential as we get older to support proper waste removal from the cells and body. Synolytics (compounds often made up of peptides) are being used to aid in the removal of these zombie cells through supplements, life-style and medications.

8. **Stem Cell Exhaustion**: Stem cells are undifferentiated cells that can turn into specific cells as the body needs them to support new body tissues, or maintain or repair existing cellular tissue. Stem cells decline as we age, along with the body's ability to regenerate, replicate and rejuvenate. The greater the damage to cells through senescence, DNA damage and metabolic chaos, the more rapid the loss of stem cells. Several upcoming chapters will review how to naturally stimulate stem cell production.

9. **Altered Intracellular Communication:** Our cells speak to one another through chemical signals. The cells live in an "environment" which can, as we age, be impacted by the other hallmarks listed, creating a highly inflammatory state. Inflammation disrupts proper cellular communication which causes impaired immune hormone and neuro-transmitter signaling along with the accumulation of AGE's, senescent cells and other waste products in the cells and body.

    Your immune system is your defense system, when this goes offline, the rate of pathology or disease accelerates in the body. Your hormones and neurotransmitters are like messengers and signals that drive powerful emotions and functions throughout the brain and body. Impaired signaling can lead to the onset and acceleration of frailty, sickness and disease, along with cognitive decline and dysfunction. While an increase in AGEs impairs proteostasis, which increases the rate of breakdown in the collagen and elastin of the skin. This causes lines and wrinkles while decreasing the rate of tissue repair and healing in the body.

    When the sources of inflammation are decreased, the body is able to slow down the rate of biological aging. From removing senescent cells and supporting cellular health, improving intracellular communication is essential for enhanced system-wide function to keep you looking and feeling your best.

As you probably noticed, each hallmark doesn't exist in a petri dish; rather, each is informed and impacted by external lifestyle or environmental cues.

Often the idea of living longer is of zero interest if it means we experience a decline in the quality of that life. This is why several of the conversations throughout this book are around Healthspan and Wellspan – and the codes that directly support our ability to thrive and express optimal health as we move through the years.

Healthspan includes the factors that impact how well the body functions so it can express health for as long as possible. This is the intersection of lifestyle and environment, the connection point between how your outerworld and daily life is directly signaling and informing your inner expression of health and longevity. This is the science of epigenetics.

Yes, what you eat and drink matter, as does how well you move, the quality and amount of air you breathe, clean water you drink, light or sound you take in, whether you are indoors or out, and seated or standing for the majority of your day. How well and how much you sleep is also critical, as is your exposure to toxins, pollutants, pathogens, EMF, radiation and stressors. Each of these factors will either speed up or slow down your biological rate of aging in the body.

Yet if these factors are so important, why, as mentioned in the introduction, are there countless stories of people who smoke and drink and live to one hundred and others who are vegans and run ten miles every day and die before turning thirty-five?

The answer moves us into our final category: Wellspan.

Wellspan is the "wildcard" – the combination of nuanced variables, unique to each individual, that create wellbeing. In fact, wellbeing has been found in numerous studies to reduce all-cause mortality and add additional years to lifespan.

Wellbeing is the objective measurement of factors like safe housing, access to resources, education, and economic sufficiency, paired with subjective measures like social connection and community; purpose; love; spiritual health inclusive of beliefs and values; intellectual stimulation (i.e. staying curious to learn or engage in new things); financial health; vocational health; emotional intelligence; and joy.

Your unique genetic code holds the key to your longevity blueprint, and the right type of sleep, nutrition, movement, environment, supplements, stress optimization and more are all available today taking the guesswork out of your health optimization. Once you uncover what is right for you, you can begin to personalize your lifestyle in ways that enhance your Lifespan, Healthspan, and Wellspan.

At the back of this book is a longevity blueprint assessment. It will give you immediate, short- and long-term insights on where and how to begin taking precise action so you can look, feel and live your life optimized.

For the complete references for this chapter visit:
www.codesoflongevity.com

MIND

Age is whatever you think it is.
You are as old as you think you are.
–Muhammad Ali

What the mind believes, it can see and achieve.

The authors in this section invite you to harness the power of your ageless mind. May you be inspired into new possibilities waiting for you.

CHAPTER THREE

Centenarian Wisdom for Ageless Living

An interview with Dr. Mario Martinez

As we set out on this journey to better understand what is possible, there is much we already know and can build upon. This adventure of breaking through 120 into new realms of ageless living will be both a culmination of ancient wisdom and modern solutions that will reveal new ways of expressing longevity.

During the 5-day longevity summit I hosted, bringing together more than 65 of today's top health optimization and longevity leaders, I had amazing conversations. One of which was with Dr. Mario Martinez. He is known for his work in studying centenarians. Our conversation was inspiring and insightful, offering proven strategies to uplevel our brains, body and being for a truly thriving, long and fulfilling life.

Dr. Melissa: Dr. Martinez, it's great having you here. You are known for your work in longevity through studying centenarians. What can we learn from them that will support us to live a long and thriving life?

Dr. Martinez: As a neuropsychologist, I was trained about the brain, how it functions and what interacts with it to create outcomes but at that time, never looking at how culture affects the brain. So there's a field now of cultural neuroscience that actually looks at the fact that the brain is not something monolithic in every culture, but the brain learns the language of the culture. And then it speaks to the immune system. In this way, the immune system is cultural as well. Meaning, how our brain understands and perceives life is actually communicated by way of the immune system to the body.

As I looked at this connection, I thought, what if I want to know about longevity? Why don't I go to where it's working, not to people that die at 30, or to people that are in their 80's or 90's and suffering but people that are over a hundred that are healthy. I started looking all over the world for centenarians, people who are a hundred and above who actually are healthy and defy all of the rules of gerontology. Unfortunately, gerontology studies the pathology of aging by recognition. I went out to see what causes health as you're growing older.

What I found in my studies from around the world is that 25% of longevity is genetics, while the rest is cultural, which includes food and everything else, but it's not just the food, it's a consciousness.

I found that these people have specific ways of looking at the world.

It has nothing to do, whether they live in mountains, whether they eat meat, or no meat, *what they are is flexible.*

If they are a vegan or vegetarian, carnivore or pescatarian, whatever, and you invite them to a barbecue, they'll go to the barbecue and they'll eat the barbecue.

Flexibility is one of the causes of health to be rigid with the things that you do is a cause of fear and fear will actually cancel out what you're trying to do healthy. So it's very important to see that.

I learned that they have a way of life. They have a sense of humor. They know how to forgive.

They're flexible, they're active. They think they're going to live forever, but they're not afraid of dying. And they know how to eat on time. Also, you elongate time, by the way that you see the future.

So for example, I always use this example because it just completely gave me an epiphany. This man was 102 at a time, and he had a vegetable garden. I asked him, what are you doing with this garden? He said, well, it's great, just wait until you'll see it in three years.

They plan ahead, looking forward to what is to come and the biology follows to a certain degree. Why? Because if you think you're going to be around forever, even if you're not, the subconscious thoughts of your brain that you have, adjust your biology. That doesn't mean you're going to live forever, but it means that you get the fear out of tomorrow.

Typically, people, as they grow older, **think they have less and less time so they compress time.** This is informing their subconscious. Now instead of thinking there is more the body thinks there is less.

They say something like, 30 years have passed and they see that as a process of aging. It's not a process of aging. What happens is that there's something called the pioneering years. These are the first 30 years when there's a pioneering of life from the first time you fell in love, the first time you had a heart break, the first time you made love, got married or divorced, all of your firsts. *And when you're doing novelty kinds of things, the feeling is that you have more time.* If you lose the novelty effect after 30 years, you've done this, you've done that, then you compress time.

Centenarians always have something going. They have a novelty effect, very high. They elongate the perception of time.

So much for time being related to aging, it's not.

Dr. Melissa: I love this. Compressing time versus elongating time, planning ahead for more forward thinking versus not enough. If you think about this kind of modern day living, there's a lot of compression, we feel like there is so much to do, and not enough time. Whether that's real or imagined. It's almost as if we are compressing ourselves into accelerated aging unknowingly.

Dr. Martinez: That's right. And it can happen at any age. If you are compressing time. If you're thinking, all I have is this time, you're living in what I call the urgent present. And the urgent present is compressing quite a bit of information, a lot of space, in very little time. And what you are doing is teaching your body hypertension and hyper-vigilance where all kinds of problems arise because you're teaching that it has to be in an alarm state. There's no downtime. People say it's stress. It's not the stress, is the compression of time that they do by living in the urgent present.

It's important to realize, stress is an interpretation that doesn't exist at all. It's an interpretation.

Studies will say crowding and loud sounds cause stress but this is true only in context.

I'll be in a culture of teenagers who go to concerts and listen to very loud performances. They have no problems. Another example is cold weather, studies show it can be a stressor to the system but again, in context. To the Tibetan lamas, they can sleep outside in 30 degrees below and they get up and they just shake the snow off.

It depends, it's culturally contextual.

This is where it's also important to look at Anthropology and how tribes get together. The culture will teach you how to get stressed out. For example, there are countries that avoid uncertainty while others have a high level of tolerance for uncertainty. The United States has a high tolerance for uncertainty where Japan and Poland, have low thresholds for uncertainty. Why? Because Japan and Poland have had invasions. They have had major problems that we haven't had in the United States. So then that culture in Poland or Japan and others will teach you to avoid uncertainty. How do you do it? With perfectionism. And what does perfectionism do? It puts you into the terrain of the urgent present.

You're being taught by your culture that you have to avoid uncertainty. You have to avoid any chaos, as opposed to learning how to navigate uncertainty.

Dr. Melissa: When perceptions and beliefs are culturally taught, where do we begin in our own mind to make shifts?

Dr. Martinez: Begin by prioritizing what is really important and shut down the urgency invitation, this compresses time. Instead, chunk down into smaller time frames, like minutes. The more the brain perceives it has to do over time, it will project and compress. Notice where you can elongate your perception. Flip your language from thinking you "have to" to "want to." Be expansive, flexible, open and excited in your thoughts looking forward instead of thinking there is not enough. These are easy ways to communicate to your body all that you are looking forward to, that will elongate time and support your system.

Dr. Melissa: You have shared so much, thank you.

As I read back our interview notes, I am reminded that Centenarians show us what is possible. Yes, life continues to evolve and how we live today is very different than those before us yet what they have reminded us is to be ageless begins within the mind.

What we perceive, what we have learned, we can evolve. Our words, our beliefs, our perceptions can be shifted into new expanded opportunities to experience life more fully. I invite us each to look forward to what is yet to come, engage in new, novel firsts so we continue to pioneer to 120 and well beyond.

Dr. Mario *Martinez is a licensed clinical psychologist and best-selling author of The Mind Body Code: How to Change the Beliefs that Limit Your Health, Longevity, and Success, as well as the psychological novel, "The Man from Autumn." He specializes in how cultural and transcendental beliefs affect health and longevity. He lectures worldwide on his theory of Biocognition and on investigations he has conducted of alleged cases of stigmata for the Catholic Church, the BBC, Discovery, and National Geographic. Also, based on how the immune system makes decisions under conditions of uncertainty, he developed a unique model of organizational science he calls The Empowerment Code, to teach executives of global companies how to maximize productivity while enhancing wellness.*

www.biocognitiveculture.com

CHAPTER FOUR

Say YES to Stress

Dr. Melissa Grill-Petersen

Stress can become your greatest ally or worst foe when it comes to living a long life well.

What does the word stress mean to you? Does it conjure up mental or emotional angst, pressure or concern? Does it equal problems? Maybe it means too much or not enough? Or, does it mean opportunity to expand and evolve? What if I told you it can actually be used to unlock longevity?

Historically, it has been explained as problematic, but I see it differently. In fact, it is actually the unsung hero of the story. If we understand what it really is, when and why it is showing up, we can say YES to stress and usher in new expressions of growth, new goals to be achieved, and exciting new possibilities to be experienced. When viewed from the right perspective, it can even extend our lifespan, healthspan and wellspan.

What is Stress Really?

Stress is defined as any intrinsic or extrinsic stimulus that creates a biological response – in other words, any physical, mental, emotional, chemical or environmental input that becomes more than your body is currently able to adapt and respond to. When this overload occurs, the system is signaled that a "threat" is present and the body is activated to "fight or flight."

This effect kicks off in the brain, sending a cascade of signals. First to your amygdala, the area responsible for emotional processing. Next to the hypothalamus that communicates with the rest of the body through the autonomic nervous system, home to your sympathetic and parasympathetic nervous systems. Finally, to your adrenal glands that activate the release of adrenaline and cortisol.

Adrenaline ensures your heart rate increases as blood is pumped to the muscles, your breath rate increases and the lungs open to increase oxygen into the system while cortisol triggers the release of glucose (the fuel for your muscles) so you can take immediate action to "fight or flight." Your brain is brilliant in how quickly it acts to keep you safe from life's threats.

This instantaneous, protective response presses the gas pedal to the floor so you have all the resources you need to handle whatever comes your way. The problem arises when you keep overloading your system. In essence, you are keeping your foot on the gas and, like any engine, unless you stop and refuel, you will run out. Your system will stop working or will begin pulling resources from other areas in the body, leading to a downstream effect. This is when it becomes catabolic, slowly wearing down the system, accelerating the hallmarks of aging and, over time, leading to breakdown, dysfunction and disease.

Our systems are constantly being overloaded in new ways, from increasing daily life demands to challenging world events, as well as others we may not even realize are contributing to our overwhelm. Contributors to this overload show up in so many ways, including traffic, video games, emails, sleep disruption, electromagnetic fields, chemically processed foods, toxins in the environment, relationships, work, medications, ruminating thoughts, and more.

Moreover, we have exchanged fighting and flighting for "sitting and stewing" – at desks, in cars, and on our devices where we engage with work and on social media. The new "threats" are also chronic, meaning that instead of happening only once in a while, they are happening nearly round the clock. To the brain stress is stress, whether it is a tiger chasing you or someone not liking a post or comment you made on social media to a person cutting you off on the highway.

As a result, the system is always "on," responding to the constant inputs. Without the proper removal and recovery, it becomes overloaded and the impact accumulates.

Being in a state of chronic distress, without adequate time for recovery, has clinically been linked to the shortening of your telomeres, the depression of your immune system, and epigenetic alterations, which as explained in Chapter Two impact all of the other hallmarks of aging.

Chronic stress due to the accumulation of higher cortisol levels in the system has been shown to accelerate cognitive decline impairing memory, executive function, language processing speed and social cognition. It also impacts your genetic expression by way of methylation and histone modification.

While this certainly doesn't sound great, a cautionary tale at best, there is more to the story. Get ready to understand when, why and how you can say yes to stress to optimize your system and reverse age.

Say YES to Stress

Stress is inherently neutral – meaning it is cultural perceptions and beliefs that determine whether we label it "good" or "bad." That said, there are different types of stress which can positively or negatively affect us in body, mind and spirit.

Eustress, for example, is considered a positive form of stress. It's a short-term challenge that gets you excited, increases performance, and motivates you to take action, such as starting a new hobby, learning a language, getting married, starting a new workout, or going for that promotion. *Distress* is the chronic stress that feels like a threat to your system. It is perceived as outside of your abilities, feels unpleasant and can be either short- or long-term in duration.

This is how to leverage stress so you can experience its many growth benefits. Short, intense bursts to the system followed by rest and recovery is the key to radically transform your performance, health and life.

This is where the belief that growth occurs just outside of your comfort zone comes from. When we get uncomfortably comfortable, we level-up our system, our health and self to lock in new gains and build resilience. This is where we become antifragile. When we move beyond our familiar zone, we are literally evolving into new expressions of our own potential.

A key study showed that acute stress, lasting seventy-two hours or less, actually stimulates new neural stem progenitor cells in the brain for upwards of two weeks. This means that a short event, followed by rest and recovery free from that stress, enhances the memory and learning of the brain.

The recipe for harnessing the positive benefits of stress calls for increased challenge or load to the system for a short duration of time, followed by rest and recovery.

That is the leverage point to enable you to experience the performance, health and growth experiences from stress. If you can embrace this concept, you will radically transform your health and life.

When you can begin to understand how stress is showing up, you can take control to interrupt the pattern or cycle that leads to distress while taking full advantage of eustress opportunities.

If you truly want to experience a more thriving life, it's time to say yes to the stress that energizes and optimizes you. A key piece of this means also recognizing when you need to stop, refuel, recharge and replenish so it does not cross into the "danger zone" – or distress.

An easy way to figure this out is by asking yourself, "Are my actions, interactions and responses to life energizing and filling me up, or are they depleting and wearing me down?" If it is the latter, it's time to pump the brake. This "brake" is the parasympathetic nervous system.

Think of your parasympathetic nervous system as your switch to rest, reset and recovery. To quickly toggle between stress and rest, engage the vagus nerve. This is known as developing increased vagal tone. This will be discussed in greater detail in Dr. Rimka's chapter but for now, know that research has shown each of the following methods are immediate tools to enhance vagal tone and interrupt the stress response. Think of each micro toggle as an accumulation of rest and recovery moments vs stress and break-down.

Meditation, breathwork, time in nature, humming, gargling, singing, socializing and laughing, massage, cold water exposure to the face, hands or body and chiropractic adjustments all activate the vagus nerve and enhance parasympathetic activity, moving you into more moments of rest, reset and recovery.

If stress is designed to automatically prepare you for action, how are you responding? Your body is giving you cues from tension and angst to an adrenaline surge or pressure to act. The more you become aware of how you "do stress" the faster you can say YES to the opportunity when it presents.

Too often, we are not aware and react vs act. When you develop interoception, the inner awareness of how your system is responding to your actions, you can start to take conscious action when stress strikes. You can begin to use it to your growth advantage.

What if you knew when you were stressed and had a "process" to toggle your system into neutral, a ready and resourceful state? This next section will show you how to move beyond the reflex reactionary response of your primitive brain and into a consciously proactive higher executive functioning state.

Here is a simple strategy for using stress as a tool for growth and enhanced expression:

1. **Say Yes to Stress through Awareness:** Notice when and how stress is showing up in your life and how you perceive your stress. Remember, you can never change another person, place or event, only your perception and response to it.

   When examining sources of stress, try to cultivate neutrality and curiosity around what you are experiencing and feeling. Doing so will enable you to more easily recognize areas in which stressors can be mitigated or used for growth and optimization.

   First begin with a general self-assessment inventory. For a further explanation of understanding how your body interrupts stress, read ahead to Dr. Leonette's chapter on tracking your stress through biometrics with wearable technology.

   For now, let's start with awareness. What does it mean and how it is showing up in your life?

   - **Perception:** What does stress mean to you? Are you gaining a new awareness from this chapter that stress is meant to be good in the right amounts and a tool for evolution and growth?

Perception alone has been shown in various research studies to either increase or decrease the risk of mortality. In a meta-analysis study of more than 186 million people, 33% believed stress to be bad for their health. Out of those who believed it to be "bad" for them, 43% had an increased risk in death from stress. On the other hand, those that perceived stress to be "good" for them or not a factor in their health had a lower rate of death, despite being under the same amounts of stress as the other group.

Consider if you can begin to look at stress through a new lens. One of potential and possibility. One of choice, empowerment and inspired action. One in which life is happening for you, not to you.

Where is Your Stress Coming From?

On a scale of 1-10 (with 10 being the highest), rate your level of stress in the following areas:

- **Physical Stress:** Begin by tuning into your body. Where and how do you notice the ways you are expressing stress? Tight shoulders, tension at your temples, unease in your stomach?

  What about forms of physical stress that you may be experiencing like trauma from an accident or injury, sitting for extended time, poor posture, micro traumas from repetitive movements, lack of sleep, lack of movement, tension, pain or discomfort in your body.

- **Mental/ Emotional Stress:** Next, tune into your thoughts and emotions. What are the most common thoughts you have? These can reveal how your mind is perceiving or responding to your current reality. Worry, wonder, frustration, impatience or joy and ease, simply notice.

Life changes can radically impact this category. Events such as marriage, divorce, work, family, relationships, love or loss are big ones. And the daily acts of being overscheduled, rumination, worry, angst, overthinking, disconnection, comparison, gossiping, perfectionism, pressure, or unresolved trauma all take their toll when left unchecked stacking up their impact on your system.

- **Chemical/Environmental Stress:** What can your daily environment reveal? Get curious about the sights, sounds and sensations that you are engaging with each day.

This area is often overlooked when considering the factors that impact the expression of thriving health. It can seem mysterious and hard to fully understand. I invite you to notice the following that you may be exposed to on a regular basis that could be a source of stress on your body: air quality, noise levels, pollution, UV and EMF exposure, alcohol and nicotine, herbicides, glyphosates and pesticide consumption from our foods. Parabens and phthalates in our beauty products and water contamination from microwaving or drinking out of plastic bottles or containers that leach chemicals, to medications and flame retardants used in many of the fabrics we wear or touch daily.

2. **Know Your Code:** Did you know that your genetic code can reveal your inborn potential towards how you perform and respond under stress? Gaining this level of personalized insight gives you an added level of support to your system

so you can say yes to leveraging your stress for enhanced health and wellbeing.

For example, while there are many genes involved with the pathways of stress, one of the most important and widely discussed is COMT, Catechol-O–methyltransferase. This is an enzyme that breaks down dopamine, responsible for the "reward response" in the brain. This gene has two main variants, one that slowly removes dopamine (AA) referred to as the "worrier" and another that quickly removes (GG) known as the "warrior."

If you are a slow remover of dopamine, under chronic stress, you can actually trigger and increase the sense or feelings of worry, unease or anxiousness in your system. Yet, if this is your code, you also have a super power within this potential. As a "worrier," you can thrive in calm environments.

If, on the other hand you are a fast remover, you are a "warrior" that has the potential for greater stress resilience, peak performance and you do well in high stakes or combative situations. You are able to stay clear and decisive while taking appropriate action. The interesting thing is you perform at your peak when you have that added surge of adrenaline to the system because it pushes your dopamine levels into an optimal range.

3. **Be at Choice:** Until now, stress may have seemed like something outside of you or things that are happening to you. Once you begin to notice how you perceive stress and when, how or to what extent it is impacting you, you can be at choice to say YES to a new and thriving state.

   Begin by consciously choosing how you want to identify and respond to your stress. This means you choose your response before it chooses you. Notice, when do you feel resourceful, resilient, clear, confident and competent vs frustrated, anxious, overloaded or overwhelmed? Which emotions feel less stressful and more proactive?

The more you tune in and notice, the greater the opportunity to by-pass chronic distress shifting into growth zones and eustress.

In the example above, if you are a slow COMT dopamine remover, understanding your code paired with when and how stress is impacting your system allows you to take control, activate your parasympathetic system to restore calm confidence so you can excel! Too long in stressful environments amp your system into worry while calm environments actually allow you to flourish. Imagine if you keep yourself in stressful situations just "pushing through" you will compromise the health and integrity of your brain and body. Yet, if you notice, and make the choice to change up your environment to one of calm, you will say YES to your superpowers. It's all about understanding it through a new lens, it can become the path to your enhanced success.

What if you are a fast COMT dopamine remover? It would seem that stress is actually really beneficial for your performance. Yes, at first glance, that is accurate, yet the downside to this expression is the longer you are under chronic stress, the increased likelihood that you will feel and experience aggression towards yourself or others.

Once again, notice your stress and be at choice to use your adrenaline surges wisely. Perform at your peak and give yourself recovery time so you don't go into extreme emotions. Understanding when and how to soothe the parasympathetic system is essential so you don't push yourself into burnout.

Some sources of stress may be more difficult to shift than others. When faced with a challenge, ask yourself WHY that particular event, person or situation is causing you stress. Then consider whether you can approach your response through a different filter – curiosity, tolerance, and so on.

Remember, you cannot change another person, place or event, only your response to it. How you perceive stress is what triggers the system. The goal is to notice when you are triggered choose this as an opportunity to say yes to what you do want and no thank you to what no longer serves you.

4. **Let it Go:** To help your system respond with greater resilience, it's time to let go of what is no longer serving you. In this case, I specifically mean, the foods, the chemicals, the toxins, the drama, the overloads to your system that are weighing you down figuratively and literally.

If stress is a natural protective system, *why does your brain think you need protection and from what specifically?* Remember, this is all running unconsciously on autopilot. By engaging your conscious brain, you over-ride that primitive response long enough to question and ask, if the items that are overloading your brain or body are truly threats. The longer your system is overloaded, the longer cortisol runs the show and accelerates aging. The faster you shift, clean your mental house and let go of all that no longer serves you, the more you free up mental and physical energy for your body to put to use elsewhere – like for DNA repair keeping you healthy and well.

Take a moment to look back at step one to the areas where stress is showing up in your life. Any item you scored a 7 or higher on is an area of opportunity to determine what is or is not serving you. What if any of those just need a quick reset? A realization that traffic is not out to get you so you are NOT under threat or that the emails are not tigers chasing you so what if you only checked them at very specific times and took a rest in between to reset your system?

Later in this book is a more in-depth assessment that will give you a better understanding of what items can make the greatest impact for you to take action on. For now, though, simply consider whether any of the above items are creating an overload on your system and what, if any, opportunities you have to reduce the frequency and amount of exposure. Doing so will give your system a chance to recover, and expand your familiar zone to include new states of health.

5. **Recover:** As mentioned in this chapter, the key difference between distress or eustress is REST. Dr. Rimka discusses this at length in her chapter. Rest allows for recovery. When stress strikes, it is critical to begin to toggle from sympathetic dominance into parasympathetic rest and reset for recovery. The more moments you create to reset your nervous system the greater gains you can achieve from saying yes to stress! Think of rest like money going into your savings account and stress as money going out. Little micro moments add up like compounding interest in your system day by day for greater thriving over a lifetime.

6. **Replenish to Rejuvenate:** Remember that chronic stress is a biological process in the body involving many pathways, nutrients and hormones. For this process to run, requires key macro and micro nutrients (the gas in the tank) to produce the necessary energy. The longer you go without the key ingredients for the body to do its job well, it will take from other tissues and organs accelerating the breakdown of aging in the body. To live a long life well means giving your body what it needs at a cellular level to flourish and thrive.

If you think back to the hallmarks of aging, chronic stress impairs cellular health and function. Proper pathway nutrients for cellular homeostasis support requires essential nutrients like B12, B6, Folate, Vitamin C, and Magnesium. This can be achieved through a whole foods diet but based on your genetic potential, paired with your biomarkers and current health expression, you may require added supplementation. Going from basic to advanced, based on the level of impact to the system, additional needs like glutathione, NAD, hormone optimization beginning with DHEA and Vitamin D3 may be required all the way up to targeted solutions like peptides.

You my friend are limitless! You are also constantly being informed by the world around you. Your life is reflecting back to you the quality of the signals it is receiving.

If you desire improvement in any aspect, take note if you are saying yes to stress and using it as a healthy tool to evoke growth and change, or if you are letting it add to the burdens that are literally preventing your growth.

Stress is a part of life, so embrace the fact that it is never going away and, in many ways, that is a good thing. The key is to let it be a teacher, a guide to show you what you want and need for your continued evolution and expression of vitality.

Now you have a greater understanding of stress in your body, environment and life. Dr. Leonette's chapter shares how you can use wearable technology to monitor your body's response to stress through HRV tracking. As you gain awareness, you can choose to reduce and remove as much "distress" as possible, then key into your eustress. Develop and train your parasympathetic system so you can move from distress into neutral to then shift into eustress for achievement, growth and expansion when followed by rest and recovery.

I invite you to respond moment by moment, through celebrating all that IS good and all that you are doing to experience the fullness of your health, vitality and life. Let the momentum carry you into doing more of what energizes and ignites you, while reducing the amount and frequency of interacting with any input that wears your system down.

When you say yes to stress, you say yes to YOU and your desire to look, feel and live your best – and longest – life possible!

For the complete references for this chapter visit:
www.codesoflongevity.com

CHAPTER FIVE

Energy Psychology: a Path to Longevity

Christina Reeves

As humans, we spend about ninety-five percent of our time operating from our subconscious mind. In *The Biology of Belief*, Dr. Bruce Lipton states that the subconscious mind is one of the most powerful information processors we know. It is constantly observing and picking up environmental clues from the surrounding world, while at the same time monitoring the body's internal awareness. It does all of this without the help, supervision or even awareness of the conscious mind, which in effect has been hijacked and running old habitual programs. We are living on autopilot.

The famous quantum physics "delayed-choice" experiment conducted by physicist John Wheeler confirmed his proposition that we live in a participatory universe. Essentially, this means that nothing happens without an observer. We are both the creators of the events of our lives and the experiencers of what we create. Both are happening at the same time!

This begs the question, "Is it possible that our beliefs and our deepest feelings manifest in our physical body as disease?" Hormonal secretions such as dopamine, serotonin, and cortisol indicate that this is the case. While DNA is certainly important and is the code that carries the language of life in our cells, there is another force that is telling it what to do with this information. This is a branch of biology called epigenetics.

As a Transformational Coach and Energy Psychologist in practice for the last twenty-plus years, I firmly believe that energy is the medicine of the future. Energy Psychology is the name given to a variety of therapies that work with the body's innate energy system to produce a physical and psychological change by restoring balance perpetuating homeostasis on the mental and physical planes. EP embraces the Mind-Body connection using non-invasive techniques that rapidly release emotional blocks, foster healing and change emotional patterns at a deep core level.

Our beliefs, both conscious and subconscious, are part of a vast information system that we call the field of energy, and it is influencing our biology. In fact, a growing body of scientific evidence suggests that it is our beliefs that hold the key to our health, to life, to our reality and even longevity!

After working with me, many of my middle-aged clients report feeling better than they did in their thirties. Most of them have learned to relax, to live lightly and enjoy life; they unequivocally feel younger than they did years ago. Our generation is being celebrated for its willingness to challenge the prevailing previous assumptions of aging. Rather than looking at the second half of our lives as a time of deterioration in body and mind, we view aging as an opportunity for renewal and revitalization.

It is true that the human body is a biological machine that deteriorates steadily over time; however, how quickly we deteriorate depends largely on our lifestyle, habits and belief systems. Psychological age is the subjective experience of how old we feel. Although we cannot reverse our chronological age, we can reverse the more important measures of biological and psychological age. We are magnificently organized networks of energy, information and intelligence constantly interacting with our environment and fully capable of renewal.

Conventional medicine, at its foundation, focuses on the biochemistry of cells, tissue, and organs. EP focuses on the subtle energy fields of the body that organize and control the growth and repair of cells, tissue, and organs. In fact, changing energy patterns may be the most efficient, least invasive way to improve the health of organs, cells, and psyche.

We all have what I call the "writing on our walls" of our sub-conscious mind. At some point in our life we will hit that wall, be in the form of illness, discomfort, or brain fog. Perhaps we realize we are simply not happy with our life and will find that we need to clean up our energy fields. This principle is explored in Dr. John Diamond's book, *Life Energy: Using Meridians to Unlock the Hidden Power of Your Emotions*. He writes that if we want to help overcome the root of the disorder, whether mental or physical, we have to raise the Life Force Energy of the patient.

The human brain has about eighty-six billion neurons. Emotions are electrochemical messages that cause thousands of neurons to activate at the same time and transmit the message to neighboring neurons. This connection is called a synapse. Each neuron communicates in this way, with hundreds of neurons receiving and sending messages up to five hundred times per second. The good news is that the brain is not hardwired, but, as Dr. Norman Doidge explains in *The Brain That Changes Itself*, is a highly malleable organ we have the power to transform!

A review of Dr. Doidge's book in *The New York Times* stated: "The discovery that our thoughts can change the structure and function of our brains … even into old age … is the most important breakthrough in neuroscience in four centuries."

Some of our most obstinate habitual programming over time have become by-products of our brain plasticity. These behaviour patterns that activate the neurons and their synaptic connections can be reprogrammed using EP techniques, thereby eliminating what is no longer useful. We can even set about eliminating a particular neural pathway.

To begin working with EP, we must become the observer of our thoughts and feelings, keeping in mind that it is our beliefs that cause our thoughts and it is our thoughts that cause our feelings. We can use EP techniques to release our emotions where they sit on the surface of our mind; however, while this will help us in the short-term the emotions and the behavior patterns will return with another similar experience.

The most rewarding work is to take the second step, go deeper and trace our thoughts back to the underlying root cause that is creating the energy disturbance within us. Usually this is something that happened to us between zero and seven years old. Sometimes it is even more important to unlearn, or to break down the old stories we have been telling ourselves for many years. Other times we may be working on issues related to trauma, which can occur at any stage of life.

EP works by tapping on specific acupressure points while recalling the specific experience that is triggering the energetic dis-ease in the body. This is not to say the body is inefficient; it has just been programmed incorrectly. While focusing on the actual event, beliefs, and emotions we are able to clear the emotional blocks, thus allowing you to heal and change emotional patterns at a deep core level. EP techniques such as Emotional Freedom Techniques (EFT) assist with this pruning by erasing and replacing what is no longer useful to you.

By working with EP techniques, you will literally create a new synapsis or destroy one, depending upon what you choose to pay attention to. Neuroplasticity shows that we have the ability to change our subconscious beliefs and, remember, it is these beliefs that create your thoughts and your thoughts that create your reality, including your physical health and longevity!

Take, for example, the fascinating study performed by Harvard psychologist Ellen Langer. She took groups of men in their seventies and eighties and encouraged them to think and behave as if they were twenty years younger. After doing this for only five days, these men showed a number of physical changes associated with age reversal. Their hearing and vision improved. They performed better on tests of manual dexterity, and had improved joint mobility. This study informs us that if you expect your mental and physical capacity to diminish with age, it probably will. If you have the expectation that you can grow younger and live longer, this will be your experience. As more and more people shift their expectations and experience reversal of aging for themselves, it will become the expectation of everyone.

Being able to control your Life Force Energy enables you to "choose a timeline" to stay healthy and live longer. If you are focused on living a long, healthy and happy life, you will be choosing a TIMELINE that is totally aligned with your feelings. You can prevent dis-ease in your energy field by staying in these positive feelings, which maintains an incredibly strong immune system. Nourishing your body and brain and cleansing and clearing any disturbances or blockages in your Life Force Energy will not only support your health, it will also accelerate your longevity goal.

Taking responsibility for your life is the first step in getting yourself out from under the clutches of the old belief system related to aging. If you believe you are a limited being, undeserving, and a victim with very little choice in life, then that is exactly what your reality will be.

If, however, you believe you are fully embracing the life you want to live, and that abundance, prosperity, and radiant good health are yours for the taking, then that is the reality you will manifest. When you translate your deepest beliefs into the reality of your world, you are literally re-writing your genetic code to living a long, healthy and happy life.

For the complete references for this chapter visit:
www.codesoflongevity.com

Christina Reeves - Entrepreneur, Mentor and Coach

Born in Toronto Canada, Christina is a successful entrepreneur, mentor and coach. Over the last 30 years she has created several multi-million-dollar companies running the gamut from a personal computer company, a real estate development firm; a retail chain of art galleries, a furniture manufacturing and interior design company to co-authoring the book, The Mind is the Map. As a psychotherapist, holistic life coach and energy psychologist, for the past 25 years, Christina continues to demonstrate her dedication to serving and empowering others to take responsibility to live their best life. She is a co-founder of Eudiamonia Center; a learning center offering extensive training programs for individuals to optimize personal performance levels which lead others to live extraordinary lives using specially designed curriculums, processes and methodologies to optimize their full potential.

Christina is an accomplished author, speaker and facilitator, hosting workshops, seminars and lectures worldwide on topics related to Self-Realization, Personal Empowerment, Emotional Intelligence and Energy Psychology.

http://eudiamoniacenter.com

CHAPTER SIX

Transforming Our Expression of Longevity
by Telling a Better Story

Lee Ann Foster, MS

"Who are we but the stories we tell ourselves, about ourselves, and believe?"

—Scott Turow

The stories we tell ourselves have a profound impact on our health and well-being. If our most deeply-held stories are those of love and abundance, we will likely thrive. If, on the other hand, our stories are those of mistrust and lack, our bodies will create stress hormones and inflammatory agents that interfere with our natural state of wholeness.

Our stories are influenced by our experiences, as well as our perceptions and beliefs. Research shows that our perceptions and beliefs are psychoactive, epigenetic change agents with the power to either enhance or detract from our health. The good news is that we can change the stories we tell ourselves to create healthier, happier lives. Moreover, our stories have a transgenerational impact, meaning that parents who transform their own stories can enhance the well-being of their children and grandchildren.

I know the truth of this, as I have been impacted by many stories during my life. I was given up for adoption at birth, my adoptive mother died when I was eight, and six months later I was thrust into a very troubled step-family. Like most families, all of mine have multigenerational stories of love and support, as well as those of violence, trauma, and addiction.

Humans have an innate storytelling strategy that kicks in whenever we experience trauma or perceive danger. Our limbic system and left brain literally make up stories to keep us out of harm's way. Unfortunately, those stories linger long after the threat has passed.

Families who experience a lot of trauma epigenetically pass on a tendency to be hyper-aware of danger. One outcome of this hyper-vigilance is an inherited chronic stress response that, over time, can lead to poor health.

Some self-protective but not necessarily helpful storylines my families passed down were: "We don't have what it takes to succeed in this world" and "The world is a dog-eat-dog place and no one will support us."

As I was growing up, I instinctively tried to distance myself from these family stories. I remember being as young as five years of age, looking out a window on a rainy day and thinking. *I don't belong here.* In a way, that sentiment was true and helpful. I was the only adopted child in the family and trying to convince myself that their stories did not apply to me.

As children we often create our own stories to avoid feeling over-whelmed and out of control. However, as defense mechanisms go, what serves to protect us when we are young can often limit us when we are older. For example, the story of not belonging that once helped me cope can now make it difficult for me to experience a safe and healthy sense of belonging; it is a story still in need of transformation.

I left home at age seventeen, put myself through college and earned a Master's in Psychology. After graduation, I worked as an Employee Relations Specialist and HR Director and offered private and group counseling.

Through divine intervention, I met and married the best mate I could have imagined – a visionary neuropsychologist focused on healing trauma and enhancing consciousness. But as I approached menopause, some of the yet-to-be transformed stories began to surface and create problems in our lives. The old theme that no one would support me skewed my perceptions and impacted our marriage and my health. As a result, I had a hard menopause and the onset of an autoimmune condition. As it turns out, this was one of the best possible setups for exposing the multigenerational storylines that were crying out to be recognized and transformed. With the help of some innovative brain training and psychedelic psychotherapy, my stories were transformed. I changed the mid-life crisis narrative to, as Barbara Marx Hubbard said, a "regenero-pause" growth opportunity story.

At the writing of this chapter I am in my late fifties. I am co-owner, along with my husband, Dr. Dale Foster, of NeuroSource, an integrative psychology practice. Each day I go to work honored and excited to help men and women transform their physical, emotional, and spiritual stories so they can feel good, enjoy life, and make the world a better place. I am also happy to say that after a lot of work using my skills as a psychologist and Epigenetics Wellness Coach, I have successfully reversed my own autoimmune condition and am healthier and happier than I have ever been. We don't have to buy into stories of fear, aging and illness. We can create more empowering, healing stories.

Here are just a few of the things I have gleaned working with my own internal processes and with my courageous clients.

Story Transformation Practices

Because our stories have such a profound impact on our well-being, one of my goals is to help clients develop their own Story Transformation Practices that are enjoyable and sustainable as lifestyle tools.

In my experience, when we simply practice being mindful of our stories, important storylines become clear to us, just in time to support our next developmental leap. It is good for our brains to have story transformation tools that challenge us to consider the bigger picture of our lives, and to improve our flexibility and compassion by considering different perspectives.

Below are just a few examples of some Story Transformation Practices you might consider as you begin to stock your Story Transformation Toolbox.

Practices for Discovering Your Stories. We have many storylines in our lives, some of which have more of an impact on our development and well-being than others. Some stories motivate healthy habits and growth while other stories may block some of the changes we desire to make.

The following Story Discovery Meditation is a highly effective way to cultivate awareness of the stories that influence your life.

Grab a journal and pen, then go to a quiet spot and sit comfortably in an upright position. Slow your breath, breathing through the diaphragm. Breathe with ease, in and out through the nose. Notice your self-talk, the phrases that rise to your awareness.

Give yourself just five minutes to stay silent and notice the phrases. Then write down the thoughts you noticed as well as any physical sensations and emotions you experienced. You are enhancing awareness, not only of your stories, but how they impact you. Do you detect any recurring themes?

Also, take note of any thoughts that felt like they were encouraging you, drawing you forward into exciting ideas. Take note of any that seemed to be of a critical or limiting nature, perhaps placing obstacles in the way of your desired forward movement.

As you practice this Story Discovery Meditation more regularly, work on your ability to notice your thoughts without attaching to them. This will help you strengthen your detached-observer self so that you experience less anxiety and emotional stress and enhance your overall well-being. (Insight, rumination, and self-reflection as predictors of well-being." Harrington, R, Loffredo D.A. Journal of Psychology. 2011 Jan-Feb; 145(1):39-57.

Discovering Beliefs Arising from Your Stories

Our stories become interpretive lenses through which we perceive and assign meaning to life events. In other words, we tend to see what we believe, rather than the other way around. If I rehearse stories of lack, over time I will automatically notice shortages and have difficulty even seeing abundance. I will then feel the anxiety of "not enough"' and behave in ways that create more deficiencies. My pessimistic beliefs will be strengthened and the cycle continues.

If, on the other hand, I rehearse stories of being in a world that is full of kind, supportive forces, I will believe that I am secure. Those beliefs will help my brain perceive the support that is available to me. In turn, I will feel safe and be willing to take healthy risks. Those supportive stories will also help me be hopeful and resilient when surprises and challenges arise.

Ponder your stories and see if you can tell what kinds of beliefs are related to them. In order to spot beliefs, look for thoughts that come in forms such as, "I am …"; "You are ..."; or "The world is …."

As mentioned earlier, my family had beliefs around a lack of support in the world, and while there is ample evidence in my life that those things are not true, the emotional and energetic pull of those transgenerational stories is strong. For some of us, especially those with histories of complex trauma, they may require a bit more work to overcome than stories and beliefs that have less history and momentum.

The takeaway here is that no matter what stories you have told yourself to this point, transformation is possible. We hear a lot about Post Traumatic Stress, but Post Traumatic Growth is just as prevalent, if one commits to engaging in transformational practices. For more information on Post Traumatic Growth, I recommend *Upside: The New Science of Post-Traumatic Growth* by Jim Rendon.

Practices to Transform Stories & Beliefs – At NeuroSource, my husband and I specialize in Neurofeedback and other brain training modalities. We think of this work in terms of dis-entraining suboptimal brain habits and entraining beneficial habits. The story transformation practices fit within this paradigm as well.

Dis-entraining practices help us clear out stories and beliefs that no longer serve us. There are many popular modalities, including Emotional Freedom Technique (EFT), or "tapping." There are a lot of free online resources to help people learn to use this powerful tool.

One of my favorite modalities for entraining new beliefs is PSYCH-K of which I am a facilitator. Bruce Lipton, the pioneer in teaching about the epigenetic power of our beliefs and stories, is also a proponent of PSYCH-K and other energy psychology techniques that address the powerful role the unconscious plays in either supporting or preventing us from making the changes we would like to make. Our unconscious contains stories, including those that were passed down through the generations, that were downloaded into us when we were young and in a hypnotic brain state. Techniques like PSYCH-K teach you how to get permission from the unconscious to accept new, empowering beliefs that are in alignment with your desires to grow.

We can also use technologies to dis-entrain and entrain story habits. Neurofeedback is one of the most powerful and safe ways to retrain the brain's habits. We offer several types of neurofeedback and brain stimulation technologies in our practice, as well as home neurofeedback options.

We have also had great success with Mind Alive, a company that offers a variety of brain stimulation and entrainment tools for use at home. Mind Alive's products are great for boosting mood, memory and sleep, and promoting peak brain states.

Create Your Own Story Transformation Practices – I like to help clients find practices that align with their personality, goals, lifestyle habits and preferences. Life is more fun when we have habits that are energizing and sustainable – and having fun is good for our health!

One Story Transformation Protocol seems to work particularly well for people who like doing guided meditations. I help clients create new self-talk scripts and record them in their own voice to playback for a personalized experience. Repeatedly hearing your own voice speak your desired belief statements can enhance and speed your self-entrainment process. You can use this personalized meditation while sitting in a whole brain posture (ankles and wrists crossed) for added benefit.

Living a long and good life requires that we learn to enjoy many types of health and wellness practices, of which storytelling is one of the most powerful. We might think of the stories we tell ourselves as "psycho-spiritual nutrients." If we habitually consume pessimistic stories, we will experience the wear and tear of living in chronic stress. If, however, we consciously craft our life stories we can improve our chances of living a long, healthy life. If we tell ourselves the truest stories – those that proclaim that we are a valued and beloved part of a mystical, brilliant universe – then we can co-create a thriving world where everyone has more op-portunities to live well and live long while contributing to the betterment of all living creatures.

Lee Ann's passion is to help people live their healthiest, happiest lives so they can make the world a better place for all. As a master's level psychologist, spiritual life coach, Wellness & Epigenetics Coach, Neurofeedback provider, certified HeartMath coach, PSYCH-K Facilitator, and Frequency Specific Microcurrent provider, Lee Ann gives her clients the type of care that is well-rounded, holistic, and evidence-based. More importantly, she helps people learn how to take care of themselves and become their own healers.

Neurotherapies, nutritional and epigenetics coaching, and learning effective spiritual growth and stress management skills have also been a great help in Lee Ann's own healing journey, including overcoming some chronic trauma and health issues. She uses her education, personal traumas, and healing experiences to offer transformational services to people who want to move beyond their limitations and become the best version of themselves.

She is married to Dr. Dale Foster with whom she co-owns an integrative psychology practice, NeuroSource, LLC. They have two fun and brilliant daughters, a wonderful new son-in-love, and an overweight, hilarious cat named Leo. Lee Ann and Dale love to take long walks in nature while discussing the deep meanings of life, absorb lots of sunshine on the beach, and backpack in Bankhead National Forest. They are both aging well and plan on enjoying the adventures of life on earth together for a very long time to come.

https://neurosource.net

CHAPTER SEVEN

Above Down, Inside Out

Dr. Elena Villanueva

Have you ever heard that health and longevity come from "above down, inside out?" If not, let me share with you what this phrase means to me and how it applies, not only to regaining your health but to achieving longevity, vitality, health, wealth, happiness, joy, and everything else you desire in your life.

What if I told you that many around the world are currently having an "awakening" of sorts? What if you were open to the idea that God (or whomever you call your creator) is not separate from you, but within you? What if you knew that you could perform your own miracles on yourself in order to heal from your conditions or disease? What if you believed that living to the age of 200, 300, or even 400 years old was not just possible, but normal and even expected? What if you believed that you held the power to create your own health or your own disease, your own wealth or your own poverty, your own happiness or your own suffering? What if you knew that you have the power to create your own experiences and that you literally are and have been creating all of these experiences your entire life? What could you achieve if you had this awareness?

Science has provided us with great evidence that the power of self-love, and how we think about ourselves and the world around us, literally creates our reality. During this time of awakening, many are realizing that their beliefs have created their realities, and that many of these beliefs stem from centuries-old constructs passed down through the generations, resulting in some very bleak and sorrowful circumstances.

Breaking free from these constructs is new and amazing territory, and it's literally creating new realities for millions around the world, both collectively and individually. If you are looking for ways in which to uplevel your healing, health, longevity, and vitality, I strongly encourage you to open your eyes and your mind to the possibilities that myself and the other experts share in this book. If you are willing to step out of your old constructs and step into your limitlessness, your possibilities for longevity and vitality can be infinite.

This is what the phrase "above down, inside out" boils down to: your mind, body, and spirit are powerful manifestors of your experiences and what you see as your reality. Your healing, health, vitality, and longevity all start with your mindset, your connection, and your relationship with your spiritual self. What you believe and perceive from the world around you informs how health is interrupted inside and expressed out.

To be clear, I'm not advising you to abandon outside information, as it can and is providing us with many healthcare solutions, including those related to brain healing and longevity. What I am saying is that your mind and your spirit serve as the foundation for such healing, for example from mental health disorders and neuro-degenerative disease.

Your body simply responds to your mind's thoughts and beliefs. Your spirit, when you connect with it, reminds you of your true self and your power to manifest your own experiences. When you realize that magnificent power within your body, mind, and spirit, and combine that self-realized power with the scientific knowledge that we share in this book, you too can experience the dramatic life transformation that millions of people on the planet are awakening to at this time.

You are not broken! There are answers and there are solutions.

This is the saying many around the world know me for. I have spent my life helping others heal and showing them that they are not a reflection of their diagnoses. Over the years I have built an amazing international team of practitioners and health coaches whose work focuses on chronically ill people who have been told they have everything from recurring cancers, dementia, Parkinson's disease and Hashimoto's to PCOS (or other "cause" of their infertility), schizophrenia, severe depression, bipolar dis-order, anxiety, and so on. These people were told "You have ..." – as if their bodies were defective – and prescribed pharmaceuticals for their suffering, only to find out that the "pill for an ill" approach didn't work for them.

While many initially seek us out because they believe we have the answers and solutions that have eluded them, what they come to learn is that they are actually quite simple and accessible. That is not to say healing happens in an instant. In some cases it can take one to two years for people to regain their health. However, during this time they start to see that for each year they continue on their journey back to health, they are gaining another *two to twenty years* of health, vitality, and longevity.

Our bodies have the most amazing ability to self-regulate, re-calibrate, and heal themselves. When the body becomes diseased it doesn't do so because it's "defective," but rather because there are barriers that are preventing it from healing. Once those barriers are identified and addressed the body does what it is designed to do best – it begins the healing process. This is not only miraculous, but a true testament to the power we have over our physical, mental and spiritual health.

Regaining both physical and mental health is key to attaining the overall vitality and longevity we desire. This is done by first reestablishing "homeostasis" (a state of balance and harmony) in the body and mind so that you have a new canvas on which to create. This is a challenge for many of us, especially those who are chronically ill and thus haven't cracked the code on what their barriers to healing are in the first place. What are these barriers to healing, health, vitality, and longevity? That is what my team and I teach to practitioners and clients around the world, and I am going to share a bit of it with you here.

Through our work with thousands of clients, we have discovered that regardless of the diagnosis or severity of the condition, the underlying causes have the same denominators. How each individual manifests their illness varies, and these variations lie in what we call the "weak link in the chain." This often ties back to our genetic code or what I like to call our "individualized operations manual," specific for the (optimized) operations of our body's systemic engines. Again, it is of the utmost importance that you realize your power, and that YOU have control over how your genetic code works for or against you. Here are some ways in which that happens:

1. There are essentially five common underlying causes of all diseases, conditions, and illnesses – the first of which is infections. When I speak of infections, I am referring to organisms within our ecosystem (planet Earth) that don't play well in our body. We have forgotten that as humans, our bodies are an integral part of this ecosystem and that when it suffers, so do we.

   Believe it or not, our physical bodies are made up of more bacteria, and viruses than human cells! In fact, without them we would literally cease to exist in physical form! These billions of organisms that help to create and sustain this form are also responsible for helping us maintain our health and vitality. In some cases, they become unbalanced, allowing organisms that are not normally a part of this individual ecosystem to wreak havoc on our body, including our brain. This disruption can cause acute issues that we experience as a fever, body aches, diarrhea and other stomach disorders; they can also cause longer-term chronic issues such as autoimmune disorders, mental health disorders such as depression, anxiety, suicidal ideation, and neurodegenerative disorders such as Parkinson's disease, peripheral nervous system disorders, and dementia.

When we have an understanding of how various organisms can alter our body and brain chemistry, and the common symptoms associated with these organisms, we can then use an evidence-based approach to rule in or rule out their presence in our body. If we find they are indeed present, we can then take action to deal with the offending organism(s) and remedy the imbalance in the system.

2. The second most common underlying cause of mental health conditions, neurodegenerative disease, and most other chronic disease conditions involves environmental chemical toxins, heavy metal toxins, and radioactive toxins. There are enough scientifically-proven adverse effects caused by these to fill thousands of pages, as they are known to cause illness and ultimately disease to every organ system in the body, including permanent alterations and damage to your DNA.

Our world ecosystems, including our oceans, are contaminated and saturated with these detrimental environmental toxins, and our planet's animal species population has been reduced to half of what it once was. Despite this data, our governments continue to allow some of the biggest companies in the world to self-regulate and, unfortunately, continue creating and using these chemicals in just about every consumer product, from our personal grooming products to our household cleaners, toys, furnishings, and even our food. In fact, less than 10% of all chemical products used in the world are regulated by government authorities, and those 10% are self-regulated based on the safety studies done or funded by the companies themselves! With half of our animal species now extinct and the human population sicker than it's ever been, we can no longer deny that these toxic exposures are one of the leading causes of chronic illness and disease around the world.

The good news is that there is now testing to identify both chemical and heavy metal toxins in the body and, once identified, they can be eliminated from the body. It's important to learn where your exposures are coming from so that you can reduce or eliminate continued exposure. I have seen the most severe illnesses and diseases, ranging from Parkinson's disease, full-on dementia, and severe autoimmune diseases completely resolve when the offending chemical or heavy metal toxins were eliminated from the body.

3. The third most common cause of neurodegenerative disease, mental health disorders, cancers, diabetes, and other chronic and autoimmune diseases are what we call mycotoxins, or mold toxins. Much like the environmental toxins, heavy metals and radioactive toxins mentioned above, mycotoxins can cause severe and life-threatening conditions ranging from kidney and liver disease (leading to death), to cancers, autoimmune diseases, infertility, massive hormone dysregulation, Parkinson's disease, major depressive disorder, and damage to your DNA. While present in food crops, mycotoxins are mostly found in high density in water-damaged buildings and homes. Mycotoxins easily take up residence in the body and can live there for your entire lifetime. Mold toxins are also known to adversely affect IQ and hormone development in children, and can severely exacerbate already existing neurological issues like ADD/ADHD and autism spectrum disorders.

Testing can be done to see if mycotoxins are present in your body, and even the particular species of these mycotoxins. They can also, like infections and environmental toxins, be

eliminated from the body. Again, it is important to determine they are present in your environment because you will
not be able to fully resolve the issue if you are re-exposing
yourself. Note that mold is not always visible and can be
behind walls, under floors, in your attic, and even in your
ventilation system, and that in the United States a typical
home inspection (done prior to purchase) does not include
mold testing. You will have to pay additional fees for this
testing, but once you understand how these mycotoxins can
destroy your health and your life, you'll see it is a small
price to pay.

4. Food is the fourth most common underlying cause of
   chronic diseases, including mental health disorders and
   neurodegenerative diseases. In fact, I have seen some of the
   most severe brain-related illnesses ranging from schizophrenia, bipolar, Parkinson's-like tremors, and even
   psychosis completely resolve once the offending foods were
   removed. I could fill pages of an entire book about people
   for whom life was a living hell because they were labeled
   with such diseases, only to find that they were being
   poisoned by their foods. Indeed, as a plethora of studies
   have shown, the foods we eat can literally kill us or cure us.
   The mechanisms by which some foods can severely alter
   our brain chemistry is astounding, and understanding them
   is critical to restoring health; however, for this understanding we usually must look outside our mainstream
   healthcare system.

   Here is a simple breakdown. Certain foods (i.e. those that
   are genetically modified and laden with various pesticides
   and other chemicals) cause alterations in brain and body
   chemistry, which in turn lead to everything from pervasive,
   chronic inflammation and a breach of the blood brain
   barrier to intestinal permeability issues.

   The excellent news here is that foods can also help us heal

and increase our vitality and longevity. While there really is no one-size-fits-all approach, testing can now reveal how our environment and what we eat affect our unique genetic codes, thus we can use this testing to really dial in on what foods are the best for us.

5. The fifth underlying cause of brain-based conditions, as well as autoimmune diseases and cancers, circles back to what I shared with you in the beginning of this chapter, which is the awareness of our belief systems and mindset and how we perceive ourselves and the world around us. Nothing has more power over us than our own mind and the belief systems that we attach to. During this time that many are now calling "The Great Awakening," a new awareness, backed by scientific evidence, is revealing how many of these belief systems have been passed down in our genetic code. Of these ingrained belief systems, some of the most common include that healing and wholeness comes from an outside source (rather than within); that aging is inevitable and brings with it the deterioration of our minds and our bodies; and that we are "old" if we live into our eighties!

As you will learn in this book, these belief systems or constructs surrounding aging, sickness, and health are simply not true. As the world awakens to the constructs, some of them ancient, that they have been born into, they realize they can actualize and manifest an entirely different reality, a new paradigm for living. It all starts with a curiosity, desire, and belief in the possibility of attaining the reality you desire. As mentioned earlier, when we understand how our thoughts, words, and beliefs affect the very fabric of our DNA and cellular processes, we see how that just as our own mindsets and beliefs may have led us into illness, they can also lead us back to health and on the path to vitality and longevity.

Whether you are just now starting your journey back to health or have been on it for a while, remember that the process of rewiring your mindset and belief system, and thus the process of cellular healing, does not happen overnight. The body can completely regenerate itself every seven to ten years, so set realistic expectations for your health and be patient and consistent, allowing time to identify and remove the stressors impeding health and healing so your body can replace, replenish and restore optimal function. Remember what I said in the beginning – that for every year you work on regaining your health you have most likely extended your life another two to twenty years. Amazing!

Health, healing and thriving requires a lifetime of commitment, love, and service to yourself. This is something that for centuries has been considered "selfish." This is another of those inherited beliefs and it couldn't be further from the truth. The ability to love and nurture others starts within ourselves, a realization that is coming as part of this new paradigm shift the world is currently undergoing. As a grandparent, I am excited about this, knowing that as we work on ourselves, we are changing our world, and that future generations will be abundantly blessed because of what we have started!

Dr. Elena Villanueva, DC – *Chief Integrative Health Coach and Brain Health Specialist*

Elena Villanueva is an internationally recognized health coach and crusader for ending the global mental health crisis and educating the public and other health professionals that mental health conditions are actually 'brain health' issues and when the underlying causes are found, the brain health conditions can be reversed.

Elena's expertise is in helping individuals find and address the underlying cause of their depression, anxiety, memory loss, Parkinson's, and other mental health disorders and disease.

Dr. V and her team at Modern Holistic Health are passionate about utilizing cutting-edge technology for uncovering the root causes of chronic illness and disease. By understanding the intricate tie between mind, body, spirit, and the availability of access to cutting-edge technology, the Modern Holistic Health team has gained recognition world wide. Using advances in functional lab and genetic data, people are now uncovering and addressing root causes of illness and learning their unique needs for optimizing their bodies. Globally, people can now have access to what is being called the future of medicine, the next evolution of what will truly become a proactive and sustainable HEALTH care model for the world.

It was through her own experience in suffering severe mental and physical illness where the traditional western medicine approach had no answers or solutions, that she developed a keen passion for the non-traditional approach of holistic medicine. If she doesn't know you already, she can't wait to meet you and start your journey of healing.

www.modernholistichealth.com

CHAPTER EIGHT

Finding Your Limitless Brain

Dale S. Foster, PhD

"If you give a body longevity – it will want a brain to go with it."

– (Adapted from *"If You Give a Moose a Muffin"*
by Laura Numeroff)

You might assume that if you take care of your body your brain will be fine, but that is not necessarily the case. As your engine of experience and the most complex system we know of, your brain requires special attention to keep it optimized. Speaking of attention, did you know that there are specific neural networks in your brain that enable you to pay attention? Did you know you can exercise and strengthen your attention networks, just as you would a muscle? In fact, everything you think, feel, and do can be traced to specific neural networks in your brain, and each can be identified, quantified and exercised. Just like you train your biceps to bulge, you can train your functional neural networks to strengthen, thereby improving your memory, creativity, language, logic, mood regulation, social skills, and even dance moves.

As a clinical neuropsychologist for over thirty years, I have performed thousands of evaluations for clients whose brains were failing in some way. As a functional neuropsychologist and brain health coach, I have also helped thousands of clients improve their brain fitness, even when their brains were "normal." As I tell my clients, you don't have to be sick to get better. In fact, your brain is your engine of happiness, and the quest for happiness is the same as the quest for optimal brain health. And, not surprisingly, optimal brain health is necessary for optimal longevity.

Your Goldilocksed Brain

My method for helping clients improve their brain fitness, health, and longevity is through what I call a personalized precision happiness plan. This involves electrical neuroimaging, cognitive, emotional, and behavioral assessments with objective testing, and peak performance training with neurofeedback, biofeedback, neurostimulation, and coaching. I call it *The Goldilocksed Brain* process. To Goldilocks your brain is to tune it into your personal optimal performance zone. When your brain is functioning optimally you can access and manage your flow states so that life is increasingly meaningful, productive, and enjoyable. When your brain is optimized you live in your Goldilocks Zone, where your present moment life experience is "just right" for pushing on your personal envelope of consciousness.

Engaging in this process involves becoming an evolutionary, meaning you take charge of your own evolution so that you can contribute to the evolution of humanity. This is a bold and very personal decision. It is you, deciding to use your organ of free will, your brain, to answer the call to wake up to what's real, and grow in your ability to show up and do your part in the expansion of the Universe. This can only be accomplished as you evolve into your personal authentic self. When you wake up to the joy of life, the cleaning up of the mess we find ourselves in becomes not a drudgery, but a celebration.

Your Aging Brain

The famous British and American psychologist, Raymond Cattell, theorized that we have two kinds of cognitive intelligence—fluid and crystallized. Fluid intelligence is the ability to solve novel reasoning problems and is heavily dependent on working memory, localized in the prefrontal cortex. Crystalized intelligence is heavily dependent on pattern matching with previous learning and is more widely distributed throughout the cortex. (We now believe that the brain works holographically, storing these well-learned patterns everywhere, not just in a single location.) While fluid intelligence tends to decline with age due to the tendency for the prefrontal cortex to degenerate faster than other cortical regions, crystalized intelligence increases with age.

In his book, *The Wisdom Paradox: How Your Mind Can Grow Stronger as Your Brain Grows Older*, imminent neuropsychologist, Elkhonon Goldberg describes the neural mechanisms of wisdom—the kind of intelligence that increases with healthy aging. A proponent of "cognitive fitness" exercises, Dr. Goldberg, now seventy-four, continues to be involved in research into ways we can harness the effects of lifelong neuroplasticity to delay and even reverse the effects of cognitive aging. He reveals the astonishing finding that, for most of us, our right brains tend to degenerate faster than our left, both reflecting and causing our decline in creativity and fluid intelligence. However, he also observes that the brains of creative people often do not reflect this tendency—their right brains remain as healthy as their left. He uses this information to encourage us to start or continue to engage in creative activities as we age to preserve and improve our brain health. Dr. Goldberg dispels the old myth of "no new neurons" in the brain and replaces it with the truth of *neuroplasticity*—that is, your brain is constantly making new neurons, new connections, new neurotransmitters, and a new you. This means that you are literally remaking yourself as you sculpt your brain every moment of life. By taking charge of this process you decide who you are becoming.

The Spector of Dementia

Historically, our care and feeding of our brains has been rather dismal. According to a 2019 report from The Alzheimer's Association, 45% of the population between age seventy-five and eighty-four have Alzheimer's Disease (AD), the most common form of dementia. In addition, dementia incidence doubles every five years from ages sixty-five to ninety. Does this mean if you live past seventy-five you have a 45%, and increasing, chance of having Alzheimer's Disease—a mentally and physically debilitating brain disease with no cure and no treatment!?

Some might read this and say, "Just shoot me now." I say, "Not so fast." Remember you are an n-of-1. It is a logical fallacy to assume a group statistic applies to you. Besides, freaking out produces excess stress hormones, which increase neurotoxicity, which destroys brain cells. So, cool your engines and put the gun away. Even if these trends continue into the foreseeable future, this calls for a personalized solution-focused approach to your brain health, rather than panic.

Dale Bredesen, in his book *The End of Alzheimer's: The First Program to Prevent and Reverse Cognitive Decline,* describes his functional medicine approach to reversing the cognitive decline associated with Alzheimer's Disease. With his ReCODE (Reversing Cognitive Decline) protocol he addresses the multiple causes of AD—metabolic issues, insulin resistance, inflammation, and toxicity. He has over two hundred documented cases where his approach halted and reversed cognitive decline. I have personally seen the power of his approach in my practice; however, I have also observed that most clients who are already experiencing cognitive decline have great difficulty mustering up the motivation to make the lifestyle changes he recommends. This brings us to the most important topic of longevity and brain health—the *why.*

Find Your Why

If you don't have an adequate *why* for longevity, none of the *whats* in this book, or anywhere else for that matter, are going to make much difference in your life. Without a good why, you will not have the motivation to do the easy things, much less the difficult ones. If your life lacks meaning and purpose, your ongoing objection to such things as calorie restriction, intensive exercise, or cognitive training becomes, "Why bother?" or "It's too hard!"

Happiness is a feeling—a direct subjective personal experience of goodness. When you feel happy, you feel good. Humans feel good, or happy, when their needs are being met. Abraham Maslow's Hierarchy of Needs categorizes human needs and organizes them into a pyramid, with our basic physiological needs (food, shelter, safety) at the bottom. Our social needs (to love and be loved) are next, followed by self-actualization needs (learning to be your unique authentic self). Finally, at the top of your pyramid are your needs for self-transcendence – these are your spiritual needs, to rise above your limited physical or ego self.

You feel happy when you experience your needs being met, much the same as when you are united with a goal. This is called a *unitive experience.* You feel increasing happiness as you evolve through the hierarchy, having higher and higher needs met. A happy life, therefore, is one of ongoing and increasing unitive experience, characterized by such feelings as purpose, meaning, understanding, insight, joy, love, peace, wholeness, healing, growth, evolution, expansion, freedom, creation, beauty, truth, goodness, grace, limitlessness, et cetera. Unitive experiences can be small, like the taste of a cookie when you are hungry, or big, like a mystical (sometimes called religious) experience of being one with the Universe.

The opposite of a unitive experience is a *fragmentive experience,* or one that breaks you apart and separates you from your goals and your wholeness, rather than uniting you with your authentic, healthy self. Unfortunately, we have all experienced a great deal of fragmentation, resulting in feelings of pain, despair, and loss. This fragmentation is often traumatic, creating breakdowns in our mental and physical health. Here are just a few examples of life situations all or most of us experience as traumatic: childhood (often traumatic), adolescence (definitely traumatic), socialization; working in a dog-eat-dog environment; experiencing the death of loved ones; and the knowledge of our impending death. In addition to personal trauma, we each suffer from the inherited trauma of the entire human race, both genetic and environmental. In fact, resolving trauma is the main unfinished business of humanity, and yours as well. The only way to resolve trauma, heal brokenness, and undo fragmentation is through unitive experience.

Maslow placed self-transcendence at the top of his hierarchy of needs. This isn't a "leave yourself behind" kind of self-transcendence. It is a transcend and include process whereby all your experience is accepted, healed, and brought into the ever-new-now, until you experience oneness with yourself and, eventually, with all beings. The "big one" when it comes to unitive experiences are called mystical experiences; they are usually indescribable because they are beyond space-time and the brain needs space-time to produce words. If you tune up your brain, you can tune into small unitive experiences at will, and eventually the big ones will occur spontaneously. This is that evolution up the hierarchical pyramid I mentioned earlier. Unitive experiences begin as an occasional state, but when cultivated as a lifestyle they are habituated as a trait, which is experienced as happiness.

The Grand Unified Theory of Happiness

The Grand Unified Theory of Happiness (GUT of Happiness) simplifies this principle into the formula: $H=U-F$. Your happiness is equal to your unitive experiences minus your fragmentive experiences. As an individual, you are being torn apart on all physical levels—subatomic, chemical, biological, and psycho-logical—and put back together every Planck second. As described in Nobel prize-winning Ilya Prigogine's Theory of Dissipative Structures, your systems are fragmenting, bifurcating, and breaking down, then reorganizing and reuniting into higher order. Unitive experience is the subjective or inner domain of this ongoing reorganization of your objective physical matter into a living being. In fact, happiness can arise just by appreciating the fact that you are alive, an ongoing unitive experience of physical reorganization and evolution.

Habituating unitive experience is the secret to both biological longevity and experiential happiness. When you feel happy your epigenome is unfolding and instructing the genes that express both biological health and experiential happiness. Unitive experience triggers the release of certain neuropeptides that course through your body, binding with receptors on the walls of your cells, causing the expression of the genes responsible for health, happiness, and longevity.

When you are pulled back together more than you are torn apart, when your healing is greater than your trauma, when you have more unitive experiences than fragmentive experiences, then and only then will you experience happiness, and its biological equivalent—longevity. The GUT of Happiness principle summarized by this simple formula, H=U-F, is interwoven throughout philosophy, science, and religion. It is consistent and coherent with Integral Philosophy (the Grand Unified Theory of everything) and Unified Physics (the Grand Unified Theory of physics).

The answer to your *why* then becomes clear and simple. You want to live as long as possible because it's fun. The difficult things then become easy because the payoff is worth it. To find your limitless brain in the ever-new-now is the most fun and motivating of all.

Tips for Finding Your Limitless Brain

- Habituate unitive experience (practice joy, love, connection, meaning, peace)

- Resolve your trauma (get help if needed, consider psychedelic psychotherapy)

- Get creative (don't let your right brain go soft with age like most of us do)

- Maximize neuroplasticity (feed, nurture, and challenge your brain daily)

- Meditate regularly (this helps with all of the above)

- Train your brain (with neurofeedback, neurostimulation, & cognitive fitness exercises)

- Quantify your brain function (get a baseline functional neuroimage—qEEG assessment)

- Quantify your cognition (get a baseline cognitive assessment)

- Set goals for your brain functions and track your progress with n-of-1 science

- Discover your authentic vocation (work for fun, not for money)

- Be an evolutionary—grow up, wake up, and show up to help evolve the cosmos

Dale S. Foster, PhD *is a clinical neuropsychologist with more than thirty years of experience in helping people optimize their brain function and quality of life. In 2004 he co-founded NeuroSource, LLC, a functional neuropsychology practice providing brain health services in Memphis, Tennessee, and still serves as its President. He holds a Diplomate in Quantitative EEG, is a BCIA Board Certified Senior Fellow 3 in Neurofeedback, and is certified by the National Register of Health Service Providers in Psychology. He has conducted pioneering research and published on neurofeedback, which helped establish the standards for practice in the application of neurofeedback for post-traumatic stress and traumatic brain injury. Dr. Foster continues to be active in the application of cutting-edge neuroscience in the promotion of brain health; he is also an experienced meditator and meditation teacher who integrates traditional brain fitness techniques with modern neuroscience. In his book, The Goldilocksed Brain: How to tune your brain for happiness (2020), he describes his integral approach to health and happiness through an optimized brain. Connect or learn more about Dr. Foster's work at* ***www.neurosourc.net*** *or* ***info@neurosource.net.***

BODY

If we don't take care of our body,
where will we live?

–Unknown

Your body is the vessel through which you experience life.
The authors of this section invite you into YOU. Discover
why your body needs and deserves your attention so that
it can reverse age while performing at peak states for you
to flourish and thrive.

CHAPTER NINE

Optimize Your Potential for Longevity

Gus Vickery M.D.

Contemplate for a moment the enormous potential that exists within human beings. For example, humans are the only complex organism on Earth with the ability to train their mammalian dive reflex. This means we can dive one-hundred feet into the sea and spend five minutes there without oxygen, hunting, gathering and contemplating what we find. We can then return to the surface and climb a twenty-thousand-foot mountain, again without oxygen support, and do the same. Now think about our incredible ability for cognitive growth and achievement, as demonstrated by all our progress and achievements over the millennia, and you will begin to get a picture of how miraculous we are. And yet, you would still only be scratching the surface.

Did you know that human beings have the potential to live one hundred-twenty healthy and high-functioning years, or even more? For all its advancements, science has yet to identify a limit for human performance or life expectancy. When you think about how much power is available to us, given this combination of time and genetic potential, it is truly mind-blowing

These potentials exist within every one of us; they are written into the human genetic code. Maximizing one's life performance is dependent upon the ability to unlock and express these potentials.

As a family physician, I have spent over two decades treating patients in clinical settings. I have experienced tens of thousands of encounters with individuals, working with them to find solutions for their health problems and improve their overall wellness. Throughout this time, I have also engaged in an ongoing study of genetics, biochemistry, cell biology, physiology, neuroscience, human psychology, and any other discipline that deepens my understanding of human design. My passion is to integrate my academic study and clinical experience for the purposes of identifying the best strategies individuals can use to unlock their potential, enhance their performance, and live long and healthy lives.

In the chapters ahead, you will learn more about these strategies from a diverse group of experts. You will find many commonalities among them, not only because they are among the most effective but because they are perfectly and intricately interwoven to work with the systems of the mind and body. In this introduction, I will briefly explore the basics that apply to all human beings, as well as a simple formula for optimizing performance and longevity.

Approximately 99.9% of the human genome is identical for all individuals. This is because all humans have the same basic operating systems and anatomical structure. Therefore, the foundational strategies to maximize healthspan and lifespan are similar for all of us; we must simply integrate them into our habit matrix. The power of more advanced strategies is realized when they are layered on top of this foundation.

That said, there is 0.1% of unique variations in our individual genetic codes, which has a powerful influence on our overall health and performance capabilities. These variations exist because at some point in our ancestral history they conferred an advantage for thriving and surviving. Understanding our unique code provides clarity about the most effective approaches to nutrition, fitness, supplementation, sleep, and many other important influencers of our health. We now have the tools to provide individuals with their unique code and the understanding of how to create a habit matrix that optimizes epigenetic expression. Precision longevity allows us the opportunity to assess your personal data, metrics, genes and lifestyle to understand what inputs to your system are epigenetically influencing your health experience.

A classic example resides in some important and foundational genetic SNPS. Your genetic code is simply that code. Letters that are instructions when activated send the information into action. Depending on the environment of the cell where the DNA resides, depends on the quality of the signal received. For example:

- APOE is a gene that provides instructions for making a protein called apolipoprotein E. It's responsible for packaging cholesterol and other fats, carrying them through the bloodstream. We each have two copies of the APOE gene, and these may be the same as each other or different. Everyone is born with one of the six possible combinations: e2/e2, e2/e3, e3/e3, e2/e4, e3/e4 or e4/e4. Based on which combination you have paired with the epigenetic signals to the system are what determine the POTENTIAL for how your body will respond or express.

  If you have an APOE 3/4 or 4/4 status, the traditional literature will tell you that you have an increased risk for Alzheimers and cardiovascular disease. What they don't tell you is **this is only a risk IF you eat a diet high in saturated fat**. The consumption of saturated fat becomes the signal or input from the environment. This then communicates and informs cellular, genetic expression that can become the tipping point over time that impairs health and longevity.

  By eating less than 5% of your daily calories in saturated and trans fats, you reduce the input, frequency and impact of the signal to the extent that just because you have the gene, does not mean that it will "negatively" express for increased risk. The power of precision health puts you in direct control of understanding the best actions to enhance your health and life.

- KLOTHO-GT is a noted gene associated with longevity and enhanced lifespan and brain function. Yet, just because you may have this variant, doesn't mean it is expressing. A simple factor that can positively signal the activation is Vitamin D. From natural daily sunlight exposure to measuring your serum levels and supplementing with the proper type and dosage can enhance your innate longevity potential.

- MTHFR is another marker that historically gets a "bad wrap." This is the gene that is involved in the critical biological process called methylation. Supportive of DNA activation and key cellular health pathways. If methylation is impaired, it is similar to gears not turning or a switch not moving on or off. This disrupts nutrient synthesis essential for energy production and genetic signaling. Many people look just at this variant, yet, there are many other co-factors that impact the overall expression of this gene. I share this point because too often we all get enticed to go down the rabbit hole of chasing a "cause" a sign or symptom, the "one thing" that can make a change.

From genes and cellular health to peak performance and vitality, no one input equals one output. Your genes, your cells, your biomarkers, your inputs and outputs should be assessed as a whole. Like Dr. Melissa said, zoom out to take into account the whole picture that comprises your expression of health and thriving. With understanding and guidance, you can make specific changes that can uplevel your entire system.

Yet, even without these advanced precision longevity tools, you can, using the basic principles, discern the best habit matrix to unlock your potential. As you integrate the foundational strategies of health into your lifestyle rhythm, you will become increasingly intuitive. Your body will teach you what the best strategies are for you, if you will only take the time to listen. The ability to listen and understand what your body is teaching you is dependent upon your establishment of a strong foundation of health.

What is the formula for establishing this foundation?

- Provide your body with the right information

- Minimize your body's exposure to the wrong information

- Make the right information as comprehensive as possible to maximize expression of potential

This is a pretty simple formula, especially when you consider the infinite complexities or the human system. However, simple does not always mean easy. If it was, we would not be witnessing an epidemic of poor health, chronic disease, and a reduction in our average lifespan.

The human body is an information sensing system. Food, hydration, breath, sleep, environment, movement, social relationships, light, sound, our thoughts, our beliefs, and many other variables all inform our system. Our mind and body then take all of that information and engineer the best possible response to survive and thrive. Most of this is occurring in a nonconscious manner. Your body is always providing you with the best version of you that it can based on the information it has to work with. Therefore, to experience the highest performing and longest living versions of ourselves, we must optimize the information our system encounters. We must become very mindful about the types of information we are giving our body to work with.

In the chapters ahead, you will learn much more about this information. For now, I am going to provide an elementary review of each category. This is not a comprehensive list, but it is a starting place.

The Right Information

Nutrient-dense whole foods; balancing fasting and feeding; optimized circadian rhythm function and restorative sleep; proper hydration; proper breathing, mindfulness and emotional awareness; balanced stress exposures and proper management of stress responses; movement and exercise; toxin-free environments; attention to lighting and sound; positive relationships; and establishing a sense of meaning and purpose. Attending to these basics provides the body with the information needed to remain healthy and resilient.

The Wrong Information

Calorie-dense, nutrient-poor processed foods; overfeeding and never fasting; insufficient sleep; inadequate hydration; improper breathing; excessive stress exposures (which can include over exercising); sustained negative emotional states; lack of physical activity; excessive toxin exposure; excessive exposure to screens and insufficient exposure to natural light; sustained exposure to addictive and harmful substances; and others. Consistent exposure to this information eventually overwhelms the human system and results in accelerated aging and disease.

Comprehensive Information

Extended fasting; heat or cold exposure; advanced breathwork and breath holds; intensive and diverse exercise; meditation; photobiomodulation; targeted supplementation; pharmaceuticals; phytocompounds; hyperbaric exposure; peptides; and more.

These strategies require an intentional and balanced approach. If utilized properly, they provide a greater depth and breadth of information to unlock your code for maximal performance and lifespan. It is important to keep in mind that they can be overdone; and, as stated previously, their power is manifested when they are applied to a human system that has already been optimized by honoring the foundational strategies.

In my years as a physician, I have observed the power of this simple formula for restoring and optimizing health. This formula works because it honors human design.

Are you ready to explore your full potential? Are you ready to find out what you are capable of in mind, body, and spirit? Can you begin to imagine what you can accomplish if you have one hundred and twenty years of life to experience in a healthy and optimized body? I hope so. You will never regret taking up the quest to actualize your potential, and the experts in this book are ready to show you how.

Now, let's turn the page and get started!

Dr. Gus Vickery *is a board-certified family physician who specializes in personalized health consultations focused on total body and mind optimization. He is also a speaker and the author of Authentic Health, released by MJ Publishing in May 2018. In 2005 he founded Vickery Family Medicine, which has since grown to multiple medical providers serving in two locations including The Clinic at Biltmore, an innovative direct-to-employer clinic for The Biltmore Company.*

Dr. Vickery offers personalized health consultations both virtually and in-person at his office in Asheville, North Carolina. He uses advanced biometrics, genetics, hormonal assessments, metabolic and nutritional assessments, and other advanced diagnostics to determine the proactive and comprehensive strategies that will help his clients experience their best health and lifespan. More information is available at:

www.drgusvickery.com

CHAPTER TEN

Life and Breath
The Epigenetics of Breathing to Inform Youthful Longevity

Dr. Mickra Hamilton

Breath is life. It is the first thing each of us does as we enter this world and our final act as we transition to explore the next experience. Breath is foundational to our very existence and the quality and quantity of the breath informs youthful longevity, wellbeing, performance, perception and consciousness itself.

The Ancients and the Eastern cultures knew the power of the breath. In fact, they recognized that disciplined breath practices served to lengthen life and to inform a healthy and happy existence. They passed these practices down to their lineage and future generations through demonstrated experience and then recorded these practices in seminal texts to teach us how essential it is to optimize breath mechanics and respiratory chemistry. In the West, where breath has historically been assumed to be an automatic process largely outside of our control, we are only just beginning to recognize our ability to harness its transformative potential. The mechanism to leverage this advantage is the science of epigenetics.

We know that how we interact with the breath affects everything from consciousness, and relationships to physiological and cognitive performance. Optimized breath mechanics and respiratory chemistry promotes enhanced cognitive and physiologic performance, cultivates thriving health and wellbeing, and promotes youthful longevity.

Modern environmental pressures and 24/7 access to a world of information and activity has created so many amazing opportunities to learn, grow, explore and experience adventure. On the flip side, it has created a change in our natural breathing process that affects our health and wellbeing, as well as the opportunity to perform at our highest capacity. Additionally, a combination of chronic stress, processed foods, unhealthy indoor environments, lack of fitness and a disconnection from nature has created a perfect storm, ensuring a performance at less than optimal levels.

The science of epigenetics (how our genes and environment interact) assists us to design personalized and precise breath programs to perform flawlessly as we adapt and thrive under modern environmental pressures. Every decision we make contributes to this process in some way. The air we breathe and how we breathe it, the food we eat, our quality of sleep, the cars we drive, the products we clean with and put on our skin, the thoughts we think, the levels of stress we carry and the chemicals/ medications we dump into our water supply, all have an effect.

Let's get practical and perform a simple breath evaluation to determine the strength of our respiratory system and establish a baseline from which to begin a breath practice that will be a game-changer on our road to youthful longevity. To begin, set the timer on your phone to sixty seconds, then place one hand on the chest and the other just above the naval and count how many breaths you take in that time. Sometimes it is helpful to have someone else time you, as just the simple thought of "How fast am I breathing?" can change the rate. Once you have noted your breath per minute rate, continue to notice the breath to evaluate breath position and breath quality, for example:

- Do you breathe through the mouth or the nose?

- Does the breath move into the chest or the belly?

- Is the breath shallow or deep?

- Fast or slow?

- Smooth or bumpy?

- Silent or audible?

- Effortless, or labored and uncomfortable?

Optimal resting breathing patterns are achieved when we breathe gently and effortlessly through the nose, moving the breath down into the belly (imagine blowing up a tiny water balloon). A small volume of air is ideal, as deep and large breaths lead to a condition known as hypocapnia or "over breathing." Overbreathing is one of the most impactful contributors to aging and plays a significant role in all disease states. It results in respiratory alkalosis caused by low CO_2 levels in the blood. This creates an alkaline pH that is higher than is ideal. Symptoms of overbreathing are tingling and numbness, shortness of breath, lightheadedness, muscle spasms, confusions and emotional reactivity.

If you experience overbreathing know that you can quickly resolve this by focusing on the volume of breath that you breath in. By taking in a small amount of air on each breath we also breath out less which allows the CO_2 to build up in our blood. This small volume of air may feel at first like we are barely breathing and your brainstem may be screaming at you to take a deep breath. Ignore these signals and continue to take small volumes of breath at a regulated slow pace. We really don't require as much breath as we think for optimal performance and youthful aging. Remember the way a baby breathes? They appear almost as if they aren't! Once you work with this for a time you will find that you have a new stillness that is peaceful and really energy efficient.

Breathing through the nose serves as the first line of defense for our immune system. The nose filters out many harmful toxins, chemicals and warms the breath to body temperature by the time it hits the back of the nose and enters the respiratory tract. Additionally, breathing through the nose allows the nitric oxide to pool and enter the lungs to benefit the entire human system. Nitric oxide is essential for longevity as it is involved in so many processes in the body. It is a molecule made by the body that allows blood, nutrients and oxygen to travel throughout the body effectively and efficiently.

Mouth breathing, on the other hand, eliminates our immune system's primary filter, allowing carbon dioxide to be released from the body in too large of a quantity to maintain optimal oxygen delivery across the system. Mouth breathing can induce or worsen sleep apnea by increasing airway collapse and nasal resistance. Additionally, it is a big contributor to dehydration which is more impactful as we age. Mouth breathing also has been shown to result in, decreased cognition and IQ and has great impact on airway development, craniofacial morphology and jaw alignment.

Breathing rate is also an often overlooked contributor to premature aging and poor health. The accepted normal rate of breathing in the medical establishment is 12 to 20 breaths per minute (BPM); however, this breath rate is too fast for ideal breathing. In fact, once breath rates are above 14 breaths per minute the body is sent signals that indicate anxiety, which results in heart rate increases, and the brain is sent signals that we are in danger and entering fight or flight mode. The ideal breath rate is actually five to seven breaths per minute, which is known as the resonance frequency breath rate. When the body breathes at this ideal rate it is called coherence and results in a highly efficient system.

If you have optimal breathing patterns, congrats, you can go to the next level by training heart rate variability and working with brain training to create an enhanced state of cognition and per-formance. However, if your breathing patterns were not optimal, or if you simply want to finetune and enhance your breath system, you can immediately benefit from bringing full awareness to your breath through a strategic training process such as the one described below. Your body and mind will quickly reward you for it with enhanced cognition, energy and enhanced performance.

Time the inhale and exhale to be relatively equal at about four to five seconds on the inhale and four to five seconds on the exhale. Don't push the exhale out, simply allow it to leave the body. When the body is ready the breathing receptors will encourage the body to take a breath, so for now attempt to keep the timing as above until that process becomes automatic. Keep in mind that constantly focusing on the breath by using prescriptive strategies for a desired outcome or being concerned about not getting enough oxygen is another indicator that you may be "Doing the breath rather than Being the breath."

If you are feeling like you are experiencing symptoms of oxygen debt, know that we take in plenty of oxygen in a small breath and instead encourage the body to relax and slow down a bit. If it is difficult to breathe in through the diaphragm it may be easiest to lie down on your back, placing a hand on the belly so that the pressure of the inhale makes the hand rise. Once your body re-members this process it will return to it over and over again and you can begin training while sitting up. Ideally, you should spend the first five minutes upon awakening (and before getting out of bed) setting this rhythm into the body. Additionally, it is beneficial to train this breath rhythm anytime we think about it during the day and practice it again as we fall asleep at night. The more time we spend in this rhythm the more quickly the body will become used to it, then we are ready for advanced performance training.

The above strategy is a free and easy way for us to start taking the reins of gene expression through the cultivation of ideal speed, position and rhythm of breathing. This in turn allows us to align and integrate our human systems, which creates a state of optimized and enhanced performance. For the Techies and high-performance junkies out there, there are also advanced technologies and strategies that allow us to identify the uniqueness of how life has patterned into the current expression of our nervous system. Once this is identified we can get to optimizing and enhancing our performance in all areas of life! Whichever method we use, breath training promotes a state of breath, heart, brain and mind coherence in which we know who we are, what we are and how we serve; we also understand that we are free to explore our limitless potential within this life experience.

Dr. Mickra Hamilton *is Co-Founder and CEO of Apeiron Zoh Inc, a Precision Performance Ecosystem that Curates Limitless Life. A decorated retired colonel, Hamilton spent thirty years in the USAFR as a Systems Strategist and Human Performance Subject Matter Expert. She works with data-driven precision for a complex systems approach to optimize human and corporate performance. Her work as a creative disruptor in the field of Precision Performance creates a new paradigm of what is possible for human and organizational flourishing.*

www.ApeironZoh.com

CHAPTER ELEVEN

Preconceive Longevity

How Fertility, Diabetes, and Longevity are Related: Reversing Type F Diabetes in the Primemester

Dr. Cleopatra Kamperveen

What becomes possible for us when our longevity is addressed *before* we are even conceived?

This revolutionary question is at the heart of this chapter and my body of work.

It all starts with the primemester™. Before I explain what I mean by the primemester, I want to put this question into context for you.

In 1978, my beautiful twenty-seven-year-old mother passed away giving birth to me. Her death was deemed preventable and the result of poor healthcare. My mother was a woman of color and a new American who spoke little English. Four decades later, this reality is still faced by Brown and Black women every day.

From that beginning, as you might imagine, I possessed a deep understanding of reproduction as one of the most important things in the world by the age of six. I also became preoccupied with a very large question that was so far beyond my years: "What can I do to help to ensure that reproduction goes well for as many women, children, and families in the world as possible?"

One month after my eighteenth birthday, I formally began my life's work in a pregnancy laboratory, where I started developing what is now known as the Primemester Protocol™. As part of the first generation of formally educated females in my family, I worked harder than seemed humanly possible, and overcame all odds, to get a PhD. I completed my doctoral training in health and social psychology and statistics, as well as postdoctoral training in social epidemiology, population health, and human development and aging. In 2010, at the age of thirty-one, I became the first woman of color in history to be hired on the tenure-track in the Leonard Davis School of Gerontology at the University of Southern California—the oldest and largest school of gerontology in the world.

Specializing in fertility, pregnancy, and the intergenerational transmission of health, I did not appear to fit well—and, in fact, was largely ostracized—in a school focused on aging. However, as a result of my scientific research, life history, and practice helping couples overcome fertility challenges and reproductive aging to have their superbabies, I approached this work from a different perspective. I understood that the health and aging of one generation are merely a continuation of the health and aging of the previous generation, and precursors to the health and aging of coming generations—unless that continuum is actively intercepted. In fact, in 2013, I introduced a revolutionary idea to the aging and human development scientific literatures: that aging begins before birth. In fact, aging actually begins *before* conception. And the key to aging, at every and any stage, is epigenetics.

Epigenetics is a Greek word whose literal translation is "above genetics." Epigenetics refers to the process through which the expression of certain genes can be activated or suppressed through how you interact with each twenty-four-hour period and season, how you sleep, what you think and worry about, what you consume and surround yourself with, how you move your body, and how you connect with other beings and nature.

What this means is that your genes are not your destiny—especially if you can account for your unique DNA in how you take care of yourself, including your biological clock and fertility. Through epigenetics, you have the power to shape how your genes express themselves to produce your fertility, health, and longevity. Similarly, through epigenetic inheritance, you can shape your children's and grandchildren's fertility, health, and longevity so that they have better experiences than you saw unfold in your parents and grandparents.

At The Fertility & Pregnancy Institute, we use "primemester epigenetics" to overcome fertility challenges, to slow and reverse reproductive aging, and to create superbabies and super grand-babies. The primemester is the 120-plus days leading up to conception, and it is one of the most important and valuable windows of opportunity that we will ever have as human beings. It is during this window when we can literally change the quality and expression of the genes that we will pass down to our children and grandchildren.

Now, I'm going to share an important new discovery: how fertility, health (specifically, diabetes), and longevity are related.

As it turns out, the reason reproduction matters is so much bigger than having babies even—which, in my world—is everything.

Reproduction is considered the most stringent indicator of health between and within populations. This is the reason why disparities show themselves first in reproduction—as was the case for my mother. However, what has been overlooked until now is that reproduction is also one of the most stringent indicators of health between and within *individuals*. Let me explain.

Most people don't know that there are intimate ties between our reproductive capacity and our capacity for living a long, healthy life. And these interrelated capacities get patterned across gen-erations, largely through epigenetics and epigenetic inheritance.

In fact, you were an immature egg in your mother's ovary when *she* was just a twenty-week-old fetus in your grandmother's womb. This intrauterine environment that you and your mother shared began to condition your own future fertility, health, and longevity.

Over my twenty-four years of scientifically studying tens-of-thousands of women and families, I discovered something that had never been discovered before: type F diabetes.

The constellation of pathologies that leads to type 3 diabetes, also known as Alzheimer's, in the sixth decade of life is the same constellation of pathologies that leads to the development of type 2 diabetes in the fourth decade of life. Critically, by the sixth, and even fourth, decades of life, we've already lost precious time and plasticity. But this isn't the new discovery.

The part that no one has ever uncovered before is that this same constellation of pathologies is already operating by the second and third decades of life, showing up as fertility challenges in both males and females. This is type F diabetes.

Today fertility is treated as symptoms. The symptoms are suppressed just enough for a woman/man/couple to have a baby. Though this result is enormous, the approach is insufficient as it completely ignores the underlying pathologies, which—if not intercepted—will continue to wreak havoc on her healthspan, brainspan, and lifespan—and that of her children and grandchildren.

We can reverse type F diabetes in the primemester and, in the process, prevent type 2 and type 3 diabetes. Not only is the primemester the answer to climbing rates of fertility challenges and conditions of subfertility in the modern world, it is also the tool for reversing the type 2 and 3 diabetes epidemics that we now face as a human race.

Stress of various forms will increase your cortisol and glucose levels contributing to type F diabetes. The most essential place to begin is to soothe your parasympathetic nervous system, reduce stressors and know that having the family of your dreams is possible.

The answer to a healthy, bright future and planet is so simple: primemestering before making our superbabies.

Or, as Dr. Melissa said: [Primemester for 120 days *before* making your superbabies so that they get to live for at least 120 years.] One hundred and twenty days is nothing to give for 120 years!

Dr. Cleopatra Kamperveen is *The Fertility Strategist. She is the Founder and President of The Fertility & Pregnancy Institute and the Global Type F Diabetes Association. She is the scientist and university professor who pioneered the field of fertility biohacking and creating superbabies. To date, Dr. Cleopatra has scientifically studied tens of thousands of women and families and has helped women in twenty-one countries on six continents conceive and deliver healthy babies; she has also been cited in over 1,000 studies in the past five years alone. She has received nearly $3 million in grant funding from multiple arms of the National Institutes of Health, the National Science Foundation, the National Institute on Standards Technology, and private foundations, including the Robert Wood Johnson Foundation. Dr. Cleopatra is the recipient of the 2020 Most Courageous award from the Mindshare Collaborative for changing the face of fertility, and she is a selected member of the Fulbright Specialists Roster.*

Her forthcoming book details the best-kept fertility secret, the Primemester™ Protocol, which she has developed and refined over the past twenty-four years. Dr. Cleopatra teaches women to use the primemester — the magical and powerful window of opportunity before pregnancy when we literally have the power to change the quality and expression of the genes that we pass down to future generations. The Fertility & Pregnancy

Institute combines this science-driven, big-hearted method with the cutting-edge process of Fertility Epigenetic Tailoring to support women in their twenties, thirties and forties in reversing reproductive aging; get pregnant quickly and easily; reduce miscarriage risk; and finally have the superbaby™ they have been dreaming of for as long as they can remember. Dr. Cleopatra and her husband Jaïr have three superbabies, each conceived on the first try using the Primemester Protocol and all born in March, right before Dr. Cleopatra's thirty-fifth, thirty-seventh and fortieth birthdays.

https://fertilitypregnancy.org

CHAPTER TWELVE

Rest – The New Four-Letter Word?

Dr. Stephanie Rimka

"Men who are unhappy, like men that sleep poorly, are always proud of the fact."

–Bertrand Russel

For years, being unhappy, low on sleep, overscheduled, and chronically busy was my winning formula as a highly sought-after holistic brain specialist. In my practice, I focus on addressing the root cause of mental illness, learning disorders, and lifestyle diseases. I take on the "throw away" cases in mental health that no one else wants; I am often the "last resort" for severe brain-based disorders such as dissociative identity breakdowns, suicide attempts, personality disorders, vaccine injuries, and Autism.

Knowing my patients walk into my front door with a long history of healthcare failures, little to no hope, and few, if any, other options, I take my role as the "Hail Mary pass" very seriously. I am also motivated by the sobering memory of how these conditions affected me. My own family and childhood are littered with the shocking consequences of unregulated mental illness, which created in me a near-obsessive commitment to serve. However, pushing myself to find solutions where none existed came at a high cost. I never saw how empty my tank was because society rewarded me for not sleeping, not resting, and never taking a break. I was praised for my hustle and grind, and the idea of admitting I was tired and needed to rest filled me with shame. So I hid the desire to slow down and continued to push myself to do more.

Rest is the New Four-Letter Word

When reviewing a care plan with a client, I receive more shock from suggesting they take a nap than if I dropped a series of F-bombs. In our modern paradigm that glorifies an addiction to work and busyness, rest is judged as weak or lazy, instead of essential and sacred. Given my passion for Special Needs children, my waiting room is filled with parents visibly aging faster than their counterparts. They shame themselves for "never doing enough." Their bodies run on stress chemicals, and their lives are dictated by a never-ending task list, an appointment-filled calendar, and a fear of breaking and failing their children. After seeing this pattern repeatedly, I realized that these parents looked and sounded a lot like who I was hiding inside.

My patients were the mirror of my own addiction to stress and denial of my inner knowing that to be more I needed to do less. I could clearly see how treating rest like a four-letter word was destroying their lives. At home, my own son was held hostage to a brain riddled by pathogenic infection and inflammation. Homeschooling became necessary, and my life quickly became about treatments and therapies to bring about his recovery. I realized I was staring into my very-near future of collapse if I did not give myself permission to rest, know, and heal thyself. It was at this moment that the Rest Revolution was born.

I knew the most effective way to leverage health and longevity was to disrupt this cultural shame pattern around rest, give myself and my patients permission to recover, and return to basic laws of nature. The principles are simple, easy, low cost, and effective.

Rest is an undervalued and underutilized variable in longevity that needs our attention. To cure the exhaustion and accelerated aging crisis, we look outside ourselves for sophisticated therapies and "biohacks," never realizing that our bodies ARE the technology we can upgrade by respecting ancient traditions of connecting to the earth. Human biology mimics planetary ecology: both systems improve and optimize through a system of stress-recovery response, and leveraging this relationship is the key to longevity.

Biological stress, such as exercise and fasting, promotes longevity by stimulating a group of enzyme proteins called sirtuins, which help package and repair the DNA. The magic, however, is not in the stress, but in the recovery. Recovery encompasses a variety of factors, including a return to the laws dictated by nature (sleep, fasting, cold, relationships, breathing, sunlight). Just as the Earth upgrades if allowed to rest after every major stress such as wildfires, we can unlock the hidden information in the genome by honoring these laws and our inherent connection to them.

Know Thyself Through Rest to Live Longer

Researchers easily make the connection between constant motion and socioeconomic stress to shortened lifespans. I suggest you can improve longevity by doing the opposite: being still and revering rest. To heal thyself from my addiction to "cerebral congestion," I chose to go inside and do less. To heal thyself, you must know thyself. Any discussion of longevity from the macro to the micro arrives at the same conclusion: self-knowledge is key to a long and happy life.

At the macro level, seeking self-knowledge is about cultivating an honest relationship with yourself. Self-awareness leads to authentic choices and intimate relationships, and fosters connection to community. Developing a balanced self-image requires insight attained through stillness. Creating a better relationship with yourself is the only way to build deep and meaningful connections with others. I wasn't capable of admitting my fatigue because I bought into society's belief that rest was for "losers." I was playing by a script that I neither wrote nor liked. Although I knew time spent eating meals with others is a known contributor to lifespan and that loneliness may be the greatest threat to longevity, I preferred to stay hidden. But this was costing me.

The human brain appears to use downtime to know thyself through a resting-state network associated with daydreaming, also known as the default mode network (DMN). Various studies show that daydream rest is critical for the brain to integrate. This resting brain state upgrades the brain in more complex ways than conscious thought to establish learning, identity, behavior, ethics, and creativity; daydreaming may be the source of "a-ha" moments that inspire and advance society. Indeed, daydreaming became a game-changer for me in solving the toughest clinical puzzles in my practice; once I let my DMN take over by scheduling daydreaming daily, I no longer "worked" to find solutions.

At the micro level, the cell must continue to self-identify and remember who it is to maintain youth and enhance longevity. The ability to remember "who it is" is determined by the health of your DNA. The greatest threat to a cellular identity crisis and increased biological aging is damage to the chromosome containing your DNA. We need biological stress to thrive and live long. However, there is a point at which stress provides diminishing returns. Inside a cell, if you break the chromosome, you can quickly die or develop cancer, for instance. Therefore, prevention of damage and excellent repair to the chromosome is critical for a cell to remember "who it is" and age well.

Sleep and Nature Cycles

As mentioned earlier, rest includes sleep/napping as well as "waking rest" such as meditation, daydreaming, fasting, and being in nature and receiving all she gives. The importance of sleep cannot be stressed enough, and the benefits too numerous to list; suffice it to say that when it comes to longevity, the appropriate quantity and quality of sleep leads to an incredible ROI.

If you want to live a long life well, prioritize your sleep. The literature all concludes 7-9 hours a night is what is needed for everyone. Based on genetics you may do well with less sleep which means 7-8 hours or you may need more which means 8-9 hours yet nowhere does the research show physical or cognitive health and peak performance with chronically lower or elevated amounts. If you try to push it to squeeze in more tv, emails, or activities each night getting only five or six hours instead of prioritizing your sleep the impact accumulates, and has significant consequences:

- One night of sleeplessness causes a decrease in DNA repair gene expression and an increase of DNA breaks.

- One night of partial sleep deprivation in people over 60 causes changes associated with biological aging, including but not limited to increased gene expression indicative of DNA damage.

I suggest you think of sleep as part of a larger context that includes your waking hours – in other words, as a twenty-four-hour cycle rather than just a six- to ten-hour cycle. It is then possible to correlate the twenty-four-hour cycle to the yearly cycle of the earth; for example, the day/night rhythm can be seen as the summer/winter rhythm. Therefore, when considering ways to optimize sleep we must look beyond hormones such as melatonin, human growth hormone, and cortisol to the effects of winter on the body, since each night your body essentially experiences a "metabolic winter."

What happens during winter? You are cold, and you don't eat very much. This is why sleeping in the cold on an empty stomach turns on longevity genes! The twenty-four-hour sleep cycle viewpoint helps us to understand how our brainwaves, DMN, hormones, food deprivation (fasting), cold stress, sunlight, artificial light, electromagnetic fields, and ketosis can be leveraged through "waking rest" activities to support sleep and longevity.

What you do during the day in the light affects how you will perform during the night in the dark.

Regulating sleep isn't just about making sure your room is dark and cool with no lights or sounds from devices. It isn't just about ending your eating window 2-3 hours before sleep to move into a fasted state or ensuring you are not consuming sugars or caffeine that will interfere with normal hormone cycles. It's not just about breathing mechanics for proper oxygen saturation, it's this and so much more. When you step back and view the entire 24-hour cycle you can begin to see the opportunities available all day long to support deep, restorative sleep. The earlier in the day you begin, the better you will sleep at night.

Rest Beyond Sleep

Meditation is an efficient waking rest activity. Telomeres, the end cap of chromosomes, play a large role in aging via accelerated shortening. A few studies have found that meditation increases telomere length and protects your DNA. Experienced meditators also have less inflammation by silencing two pro-inflammatory genes: RIPK2 and COX2. In addition, the extent to which these genes were silenced translated to a faster cortisol recovery test, implying an increase in resiliency after stress.

Fasting is an important side effect of sleep time. Calorie-restriction is consistently shown to increase longevity – the trick is to utilize hunger just enough to initiate longevity pathways without causing starvation damage. Fasting is also another form of rest for the body, as it avoids eating and digestion during this time. An easy way to extend winter-ketosis-sleep benefits is to fall asleep on an empty stomach, skip breakfast occasionally during the week, and add one twenty-four to seventy-two-hour water fast each month.

Unfortunately, there is not much research surrounding nature's impact upon epigenetic expression. However, one study did examine how urban environments may increase mental health problems by DNA methylation changes. In another interesting study, researchers investigated the epigenetic effects of urbanism comparing the farming Bantu with that of the hunting-gathering Pygmies. The authors found epigenetic differences leading to gene mutations that are hereditary due to long-term lifestyle differences. They concluded that the results suggest living in cities away from nature has an "influence on the susceptibility to immunity-related disorders, as previously hypothesized for allergies and inflammatory bowel disease."

Nature immersion may very well connect the code of the human design, serving as the "technology" across all variables in longevity. Living in direct connection with the cycles of the earth and seasons, our physiology is naturally directed into a proper twenty-four-hour sleep cycle with built-in stress/rest-recovery adaptations from sunlight/dark cycles, cold and heat stress, daily and seasonal fasting, proper breathing cycles, exercise, idle time, and balanced exposure to native versus non-native electromagnetic fields. An emerging field called ecopsychology is attempting to demonstrate how simply being in natural environments affects brain performance by improving tasks such as memory, learning, and creativity.

All the data around longevity suggests that a Rest Revolution is long overdue.

We have an inherent need to rest in nature. Addiction to constant productivity is costing us lifespan, but returning to lessons learned from nature can help us remember we are the most advanced technology ever designed. Biological stressors such as exercise and fasting are only effective if they are balanced with adequate recovery for an upgraded longevity response. By culturally destroying reverence for rest, we are not accessing our epigenetic power to thrive as we age. You may be able to increase your lifespan through medications, but what is the quality of those extra years? Giving your brain and body permission for downtime allows it to heal DNA damage, lengthen telomeres, regulate hormones, activate the DMN, integrate self-identity, and breathe properly; this increases your healthspan. Accepting that rest is not a luxury, but rather a necessity, also helps us ward off feelings of shame, isolation, and loneliness, which destroy all sense of wellspan.

You can leverage the power of stress-recovery by spending fifteen minutes per day doing absolutely nothing, preferably while outside, immersed in nature. And "nothing" means NOTHING: no music, chanting, meditation, walking, planning, et cetera. Do this for thirty days and be amazed at the revolution inside that rest creates.

Dr. Stephanie Rimka, BA, DC, BCN *is a holistic brain optimization specialist focused on integrated neurotherapies to identify and address the root cause of mental illness, learning disorders, and chronic illness. She utilizes 19-channel QEEG brain imaging and addresses genetic implications in emotional trauma, somatic translation of illness, and mental illness. Dr. Rimka is the winner of the People's Choice Award 2020 for Best Mental Health Practice in Buckhead via Atlanta Best Media Group. She graduated from Albion College, Albion MI 1995 (BA); Life University, Atlanta, GA, 2000 (DC); BCIA certified (BCN); Wahls Protocol certified; Scientific Advisory Board Member for New U Life Corporation; CEU Certified Chiropractic Instructor State of GA.*

In addition to her private practice, Dr. Rimka teaches courses in her e-learning center, leads healing retreats internationally, teaches colleagues, and, most importantly, spends time with her teenage son, Bennett. She loves motorcycles, tropical beaches, bonfires, and group experiential learning. **https://brainandbodysolutions.com**

CHAPTER THIRTEEN

Energize Your Cells

Male 2.0 a Systems-Based Approach to Reverse the Aging Process

Tracy Gapin, M.D.

Fred, a high-level executive, came into my office complaining of fatigue, difficulty focusing at work, and low libido. His mind wasn't as sharp as it used to be, and he sometimes had trouble concentrating to the point that it affected his job performance. The most frustrating thing, however, was his weight, which had gradually crept up despite the fact that he had been following the keto diet religiously. When Fred researched his symptoms, he found several articles suggesting that his testosterone levels might be off, and that I might be able to "fix" him with a shot.

When I ran labs on him, I found that, indeed, Fred's testosterone level was that of a man in his eighties. The problem was, he had recently turned forty-five!

I would like to say I was shocked, but the truth is I see men like Fred every day. They are in the prime of life, yet they feel like men their father's age could run circles around them. They feel betrayed by their own bodies.

The good news is that we've made incredible progress in the fields of health optimization and longevity, meaning we're not only able to combat the symptoms of aging like Fred is experiencing, but actually reverse the aging process. We understand that while our testosterone level is important, it's only one part of the equation. Our bodies are a magnificent network of interrelated systems, hormones, neurotransmitters, and other key enzymes; therefore, we can't expect to optimize our health or extend longevity by simply focusing on one aspect. Instead, we need to take a comprehensive, holistic approach, focusing on every aspect of the human system.

As a board-certified urologist and men's health expert specializing in precision medicine, I've helped thousands of patients regain their energy, focus, and vitality, helping them function better than they have in years, sometimes decades. Along the way, I also transformed my own health.

In my forties, I found myself in the same position as many of my patients – sluggish, fatigued and lacking my former zest for life. I was overweight, stressed out, not sleeping well, not exercising, and feeling like crap. Worse yet, I found there was very little in the way of answers from my traditional primary care physician. His bland, tone-deaf suggestions to simply eat more vegetables, exercise more, and maybe take a statin did not sit well with me.

This served as a catalyst, not only to take charge of my health but also to shift the paradigm of men's health in general. I'm no longer focused on simply treating disease or stamping out symptoms, but on optimizing lifespan (how long we live) and, just as important, healthspan (how *well* we live). To accomplish this, we need to overcome the hallmarks of aging discussed earlier in this book by focusing on three key targets:

- Optimizing cellular efficiency

- Mitigating cellular damage

- Optimizing hormone levels

Optimizing Cellular Efficiency

Cellular efficiency can be thought of like keeping the engine of your car running smoothly. You want all the key components of your cells functioning at their peak. We know that the aging process is promoted by deterioration in such cellular function, so optimizing this efficiency is critical.

Improving cellular efficiency starts with supporting the mitochondria, the powerhouse of every cell. Mitochondria are important for energy production, cellular signaling, cellular growth, and cell death. One way to improve mitochondrial function is to increase our levels of a molecule called NAD (nicotinamide adenine dinucleotide). NAD is an important molecule that is central to metabolism and energy production. Along with micronutrients found in foods, the mitochondria utilize NAD to create an essential form of energy called adenosine triphosphate (ATP). As we age, NAD levels decline, which leads to mitochondrial dysfunction. More research on how to best increase NAD levels is needed, but in many cases intermittent fasting (time-restricted feeding with at least 16 hours of fasting each day), interval training, and NAD-boosting supplements such as NMN (nicotinamide mononucleotide) or NR (nicotinamide riboside) have found to be effective.

Other ways of supporting mitochondrial function include cold thermogenesis (such as cold shower, ice baths, or cryo chambers), high intensity interval training, intermittent fasting, and improving sleep quality. Other supplements that effectively upregulate (turn on) mitochondrial function include curcumin, Bacopa, quercetin, and Holy Basil.

We can also improve cellular efficiency through a process called autophagy, which is the process of shedding old cellular debris to make room for the cell to function properly. This can be thought of like taking out the trash. For the cell to function at its peak, it needs to be clear of metabolic waste. Autophagy is promoted by consuming the right amounts of nutrients and micronutrients – specifically, by focusing on high quality whole foods, healthy omega-3 and monounsaturated fats, and avoiding processed foods and refined sugars. Intermittent fasting, high intensity exercise and supplements like resveratrol can all promote autophagy as well.

Mitigating Cellular Damage

Optimizing cellular function and efficiency alone won't be effective unless we also mitigate the cellular damage that occurs constantly.

One of the most significant causes of cellular damage and thus aging is chronic inflammation. It's important to understand that there are two types of inflammation — acute and chronic. Acute inflammation is your body's natural response to something that has gone wrong, such as injury or infection. White blood cells secrete cytokines (pro-inflammatory enzymes) to get rid of toxins and help your body repair damaged tissue, then the inflammatory response fades. This is a good thing.

With chronic inflammation, however, the cytokines don't go away when the acute insult has cleared. The inflammatory response persists, ultimately causing extensive damage to healthy tissue, epigenetic alterations, shortening of our telomeres, and ultimately promoting the aging cascade. A key part of age reversal, therefore, is eliminating chronic inflammation.

Another source of cellular damage is oxidative stress. This term refers to disruption of the delicate balance between your body's antioxidant system and reactive oxygen species such as free radicals and peroxides that are produced during normal cellular function. Excess reactive oxygen species damage DNA, proteins, and other key cellular structures, thereby promoting aging and other chronic diseases.

So, what promotes chronic inflammation and oxidative stress?

- Inflammatory diet – processed foods, simple sugars, refined carbohydrates (i.e. white flour), sugars, gluten, alcohol, and unhealthy fats such as trans fats and omega-6 poly-unsaturated fats (i.e. corn oils)

- Poor sleep quantity and/or quality

- Chronic emotional stress

Another source of cellular damage is senescent cells – those that have lost normal cellular function but won't quite go away. Instead of undergoing apoptosis (cellular death), they secrete toxic cytokines that damage nearby healthy cells, especially the all-important stem cells. Recent research shows that a critical key to promoting longevity is clearing senescent cells with drugs and supplements called senolytics. Senolytics currently being studied include quercetin, fisetin, and rapamycin.

Optimizing Hormone Levels

Another theory of aging centers around hormone function. We've known for a long time that as we age our hormones levels decline. It's also clear that age-related diseases are associated with these hormone deficiencies. More recently, we've also come to understand that we may be aging *because* our hormone levels are declining.

To manage the symptoms of aging as well as potentially reverse its underlying causes, we need to focus on optimizing hormone levels as we age. Testosterone levels in men drop by approximately 1% as they age. This leads to loss of muscle and bone density, as well as cognitive decline, low energy and loss of libido, so it's certainly important to focus on replenishing testosterone levels.

However, as mentioned earlier, it's not enough to simply increase testosterone levels. We also need to focus on other critical hormones such as thyroid hormone, cortisol, insulin, estrogen, growth hormone, melatonin, Vitamin D, and DHEA. Your hormones are a symphony, so in order to make beautiful music you must pay attention to every instrument.

Systems-Based Approach

It's important to take what we call a systems-based approach, meaning we look at human performance as a complex network of interacting components that all come together, react to the environment, and create an outcome. So optimizing health and promoting longevity requires that we focus on optimizing every aspect of the human system, understanding that they all affect the ultimate outcome. This concept led to my creation of Male 2.0, a systems-based, comprehensive approach to men's health that encompasses the following components:

- Mindset – The importance of our attitude and mental health cannot be overstated when it comes to becoming and staying healthy. Practices like yoga, breathwork, exercise and social connections keep us grounded, happier and able to overcome life's challenges with greater ease. A regular meditation practice in particular has been proven to affect the aging process. For one, it reduces our feelings of stress and the physiological responses to it, including that of chronic inflammation. Just fifteen minutes of meditation helps to increase the production of telomerase, which lengthens telomeres. Meditation also has been found to increase grey matter in the brain, helping to improve concentration and build neuroplasticity (the ability to create new neural pathways), both of which decline as we age.

- Nutrition – Focusing on a diet rich in real, whole, plant-based foods, staying hydrated; and getting proper micro-nutrients are all critical for cellular repair and other important processes. Note: this does not mean you have to become a vegetarian, or never have something sweet again. It does mean you should primarily consume high-quality organic foods, lean meats and fish, and cut back on dairy, refined carbs and sugars. Intermittent fasting is also recommended for its powerful effect on boosting metabolism and weight loss

- Fitness – Develop an exercise regimen that balances strength training and aerobic exercise. At first this may feel like a chore – do it anyway. Regular exercise, along with the other measures I've mentioned, will increase your strength and stamina, as well as your confidence. In fact, I'd go so far as to say you'll soon find yourself looking forward to those workouts!

- Hormones – Speak to your doctor about assessing and balancing thyroid, cortisol, insulin, estrogen, growth hormone, melatonin, Vitamin D, and DHEA, in addition to testosterone.

- Detox – This includes ridding the body of heavy metals; endocrine disruptors (i.e. pesticides and other chemicals); and gut parasites. Glutathione, an antioxidant found in plants, animals and some fungi, should be introduced to prevent cellular damage.

- Sleep – Poor sleep leads to more than just a lousy mood the next day; it actually causes epigenetic changes that accelerate the aging process. You can improve your sleep with healthy practices such as setting a regular bedtime, turning off technology at least an hour before bed, and avoiding caffeine.

Not too long ago, aging was considered inevitable. Now we know that we can not only slow it down, but actually turn back the clock!

Dr. Tracy Gapin *is a board-certified urologist, men's health expert, author, and professional speaker who specializes in precision performance medicine. Using cutting-edge age management protocols, Dr. Gapin coaches Fortune 500 executives, entrepreneurs, and evolutionary leaders of business and high performance. His proprietary program, Male 2.0, incorporates human epigenetic coaching, hormone optimization, peptide therapy, state-of-the-art biometric monitoring, and nutrition and lifestyle intervention to provide men a personalized path to optimizing health and performance.*

https://drtracygapin.com

CHAPTER FOURTEEN

The Movement of Longevity:
The Transformative Effects of Exercise on Healthspan and Lifespan

Jose E. Barreto MD, PT

As the late Dr. Robert Butler once said, "If exercise could be packaged in a pill, it would be the single most widely and beneficial medicine in the nation." I agree with this sentiment whole-heartedly. Some people think that we stop moving because we grow older, when the truth is, we grow older *because we stop moving.*

Exercise is one of the pillars of health, whether we are talking about the quality of life or the length of it. In fact, studies have shown that moderate exercise (where there is an increase in your heart rate of 50-70% you max) done continuously in 10-minute increments or longer for a total of 30 minutes daily is one of the main predictors of longevity and health. It affects several markers of longevity, including one's level of fitness, fasting glucose, Heart Rate Variability (HRV), inflammation, body fat, muscle mass, resting heart rate, and more.

The type(s) of exercise you perform is also important. For example, some forms of exercise unlock various mechanisms – such as mTOR, AMPK, NAD+, sirtuins, and mitochondrial biogenesis – that promote longevity, while others do not.

That said, exercise merely lives in the land of movement. Exercising for 30 to 60 minutes each day is great, but if you're spending the rest of your time sitting on the couch or at a desk, you are not living a healthy/active life. *To experience the rejuvenating effects of movement, you need to stay active throughout the day, not just during your exercise session.*

As a physician who is double-board certified in Physical Medicine & Rehabilitation and Pain Medicine, I am in the unique position of seeing patients and clients at both ends of the spectrum. On one end, I round at nursing homes, where I see the direct effects of sarcopenia (loss of muscle) in my patient's mobility and quality of life; at my clinic, I see the deteriorating effects that obesity, sedentarism and degeneration can have on the joints, mobility and quality of life. On the other end, as an epigenetic coach who designs lifestyle programs based on clients' genetic profile, I see what is possible, regardless of age, when you push "the right buttons."

I have developed these protocols over years of practice and across disciplines. Prior to entering medical school, I was a physical therapist and experienced firsthand the effects of rehabilitation, movement and exercise on regaining and maintaining muscle strength, endurance and mobility. Now, I combine that knowledge and experience, prescribing and supervising different lifestyle and training programs and perform orthobiologic interventions to help my patients and clients thrive and heal without drugs or surgeries. In doing so, I help people prolong life and healthspan and live without limits.

Muscles help you move and interact with the environment; however, their function and importance go beyond these obvious mechanical effects. Muscles are an important reservoir of proteins, enzymes, and cytokines, and are involved with and influence various metabolic pathways responsible for survival and longevity. Muscles can also be considered endocrine organs, as they secrete myokines, which help fight inflammation and have other important physiological effects.

Skeletal muscle accounts for about 30 to 40% of a fit person's total bodyweight. In addition, its metabolism can increase by up to fifty times while exercising, when compared with its resting rate. Powerful muscles are only part of the equation, however; if you want to live long and stay active you also need healthy bones and joints. Painful joints or soft tissue injury can limit many people from staying as active or doing more strenuous workouts as they grow older. In fact, obesity and joint injury are the two main modifiable factors for degenerative joint conditions. The good news is that exercise will help prevent obesity, and the benefits of an active lifestyle outweighs the risks of injury by the classic mile. In addition to improvements in bone density, exercise helps promote healthy joint cartilage and protects against joint degeneration.

Many of my friends and patients think that exercise will hurt their joints or cause arthritis, but this is wrong. Studies have shown that active people have no greater risk of arthritis than non-exercisers. Another misconception is that as we age "everyone gets arthritis." This implies that arthritis is a disease of aging, rather than part of normal aging. Also, cartilage is not the only structure affected in arthritis. Weak ligaments, muscles and tendons are part of the picture as well. In order to have healthy joints (and spine) you need to have controlled and full range of motion. Think of it like having loose lug nuts in your tire. It will be wobbly, and it will wear out sooner than later. The same thing happens when you have weak muscles, tendons and ligaments. But don't worry. There is growing evidence on the effects of various orthobiologics (i.e. prolotherapy, PRP, bone marrow and adipose tissue cell therapies) on joint health and function.

If you want to have strong and powerful muscles, along with healthy joints, for years to come, then a comprehensive approach of exercise, nutrition, hormonal balance, lifestyle modifications and orthobiologics (when needed) will give you the best results. This is why resistance training is important – it has positive effects on hormones, muscles, bone health and other things that will help with musculoskeletal health and longevity.

With aging there is a loss of muscle mass and decreased function; this, as mentioned above, is called sarcopenia. This loss of muscle does not occur in a uniform way; it is greater in the legs and affects mainly the type II (fast) fibers, which are used for short bursts of energy and then tire quickly. Longitudinal studies have shown that sarcopenia is an independent risk factor for mortality (especially leg and grip strength) and that strength is a better predictor of mortality than loss of muscle mass.

Other changes associated with aging include myosteatosis, the process where muscles start to get infiltrated with fat and connective tissue, as well as the loss of fast motor neurons connecting the spine with the muscles. This combination leads to a reduction of muscle strength, which is greater than the loss of muscle mass. This is why focusing on explosive, strong muscles is critical to preventing these changes.

A study by National Health Institute Survey (NHIS) showed that strength training done twice a week reduced the odds of dying by 46%. In fact, 12% of all mortality in the USA is related to lack of exercise and physical activity. Exercise has been shown to lower the risk of many chronic conditions that are the most common causes of death and morbidity, including stroke, hypertension, colon cancer, breast cancer, coronary heart disease, diabetes and obesity. Another common cause of morbidity is osteoporosis and bone fractures. Exercise will reduce the risk of falls and improve bone density. It also increases neurogenesis, improves cognitive function and prevents depression.

As mentioned earlier, exercise also positively affects the pathways known to be important for longevity. For example, exercise increases NAD+ levels, which is important for energy production. It also stimulates AMPK, which leads to the inhibition of mTOR in liver and fat cells (a good thing for longevity), and has other beneficial effects on lifespan such as mitochondrial biogenesis, better glucose (via GLUT4) and fat control.

Exercise increases Forkhead Box O (FOXO), which are a family of transcription factors (proteins involved in the process of converting DNA into RNA) that play an important role in cell survival and stress resistance. Things like holding your breath while walking or breathing exercises will activate FOXO3a, which promotes apoptosis, a form of cell death that is not only normal but vital in the prevention of cancer. Exercise also increases sirtuins, which are an important family of proteins involved in different cell functions, including autophagy (the clearing out of damaged cells), and provide protection against various age-related conditions such as cancer, cardiovascular and neurodegenerative conditions. On the other hand, exercise inhibits mTORC1 (found in fat and liver cells), which leads to lower fat gain, while increasing activity of mTOR in the brain, muscles, and mitochondria, which leads to better population of cells that are important for longevity and function.

Resistance training and High Intensity Interval Training (HIIT) are particularly beneficial. Resistance training increases expression of UCP1 (uncoupling protein 1), which are proteins located in the membrane and involved in the transfer of protons in the mitochondria of skeletal muscles. UCP1 expression is associated with longer lifespan. HIIT has a huge impact on mitochondrial biogenesis (the process that increases mitochondrial mass) and activates lipase, an enzyme that helps with fat metabolism. Resistance training and HIIT can also suppress your appetite, which is helpful in fasting and calorie restriction, both of which have proven longevity benefits.

People who exercise have longer telomeres, or the "caps" on the end of our chromosomes that protect our cells and shorten as we age. In a study conducted on twins it was found that telomeres were longer in those who were physically active. Related to telomere length is the reduction in DNA methylation, which, when talking about epigenetics, is associated with aging. Preliminary studies have shown that exercise has a positive effect on the expression of DNA methylation, as well as histone modification, another common process responsible for epigenetic changes.

To conclude, I want to give you some specific tips and "exercise codes" that will unlock their power and help you live a long and healthy life. (If you have a diagnosis or signs and symptoms of kidney, cardiovascular disease or diabetes, then exercise testing is recommended before starting a workout routine).

1. It is important to stay active and moving throughout the day, not just when you're working out. Constant movement throughout the day is a critical aspect of life "in the blue zones," where there are higher concentrations of people who live past the age of one hundred.

2. HIIT is important to recruit fast muscle fibers, increase mitochondrial capacity and increase your muscle mass ratio. Example: HIIT sprints and Tabata exercises (a type of HIIT exercises).

3. Engage in moderate and vigorous exercises since this is associated with a reduction in all-cause mortality.

4. While endurance and resistance training are both important for longevity, the effects of resistance training seem to be particularly so. This is because resistance training has positive effects on your cardiovascular system, but endurance training doesn't have the same effects on the Musculoskeletal system. Remember that stronger muscles equal lower body fat and better response to insulin. Several studies have found lower mortality in individuals who have a regular strength training routine.

5. Muscle-building affects hormones and hormones affect muscle growth. So, it is important to have a healthy environment (nutrition, sleep, hormone balance) for an optimal response to exercises.

6. Focus on compound exercises that affect multiple joints and lead to a greater increase in hormones (i.e. growth

hormone and testosterone) than isolation exercises. Bench presses, squats, deadlifts, barbell rows, to name a few examples, will increase grip and leg strength and help you have explosive and compact muscles.

7. If you are older, don't expect to see much difference in your muscle mass but you will definitely see an increase in your strength. Studies have shown that just six weeks of resistance training can increase your strength more than 50%!

8. Super-slow training, where you take about ten seconds to lift the weight (concentric contraction) and ten seconds to lower the weight (eccentric), is another way to improve your muscle mass ratio.

9. Isometric exercises (where muscle is contracting but there is no movement) can help with mitochondrial biogenesis and reduce risks for injury. Examples: wall squats and planks.

10. Walk while combining slow nasal breathing and holding your breath to improve muscle endurance.

11. Don't forget to stretch and participate in techniques to improve the health of your soft tissue and fascia that connect your muscles, nerves and blood vessels. This is extremely important for health and longevity.

Dr. Jose E. Barreto *is an epigenetic life coach and physician double-board certified in Physical Medicine & Rehabilitation (PM&R) and Pain Medicine.*

It was a fastball down the middle of the plate that started Dr. Barreto on this amazing journey. While playing baseball at age fifteen, he took a big swing and hurt his back. It was during his therapy sessions that he began developing a special admiration for and interest in the medical field and its professionals. This led him to become a physical therapist (PT) and eventually a physician.

After receiving his medical degree from Ponce Health Sciences in Puerto Rico, Dr. Barreto completed a residency in PM&R at UT Southwestern Dallas, followed by a fellowship VCU-Richmond, the only ACGME-accredited fellowship in the U.S. that combines Pain and Regenerative Medicine.

Every year he travels to Honduras, where he treats patients using prolo-therapy and teaches physicians from around the world in these injection techniques.

Dr. Barreto recently opened his own practice, Regenomics, in Orlando, Florida. In addition to epigenetics and life coaching, he is passionate about protecting the environment.

https://regenomics.me

CHAPTER FIFTEEN

The Wisdom Within Your Gut

Dr. Amanda Krueger

Like so many of us, I learned to unlock my wisdom within while seeking answers to a health crisis that seemed to take my body by storm. By the time I was nineteen I had a myriad of symptoms that left me feeling overwhelmed, alone, and terrified. I was extremely sick, with constant headaches, constipation that lasted for weeks at a time, and abdominal pain so severe I would pass out. I also had horrible reactions to medications, and fatigue that was in-de-scribable.

I was referred to specialist after specialist, but none could provide me with anything resembling a meaningful explanation. When the tests yielded no answers, they suggested I go on antidepressants, which was ironic because depression was the only symptom I had *not* experienced. Though I was desperate for relief I just knew this was not a solution or even an option for treatment. It would be my first experience listening to my gut, what I call the "wisdom within."

We are by design housed with this gut feeling, and our journey, with regard to our health and life in general, is learning how to understand and listen to it. As we do, we naturally begin to shift from the disease model of our current healthcare system to one of prevention and true optimization.

For me, walking this journey meant I no longer chased "symptom free" and instead focused on complete wellbeing. At the beginning of this process I was an EMG tech for a neurologist and was taking undergraduate pre-med classes, where I started to learn a lot about the science of the body. By the time I was twenty-two I had enrolled and completed a year of graduate work at Logan College of Chiropractic. This is where I really started to put the pieces of my health together. I started to understand what my body was telling me and compare that to the mechanisms of physiology. As I learned about how the digestion system worked, I began to understand how my system was not healthy, and begin taking a step-by-step approach that would allow my body to heal. I went gluten-free, started to eliminate processed foods, went on a liver cleanse, and supported my digestion with enzymes, HCL, and probiotics. The process was a little overwhelming at first, but within weeks I started to reap the benefit of my good choices. The wisdom within was now having a different conversation – one of more energy, no headaches, increased bowel movements, and better sleep. I was walking in alignment with my body's design, and it was re-sponding with improved health and wellbeing.

For the last fifteen years I have dedicated my life to understanding the different systems of the body and walking patients through their challenges and toward their best health possible. Education is my go-to tool, but I stress that in order to truly optimize their health they need to listen to their inner voice, understand their own unique system, and perhaps most importantly, be patient with themselves. Learning to do this is a process and journey, and our success often lies in accepting our differences and inherent strengths and weaknesses. What works for one person will not necessarily work for another, which is why understanding your wisdom within is so important. Think of it as your user's manual for optimized health, and one that will help you crack your personal code to longevity.

When working with patients I find it very important to discuss their digestive system and how it functions and potentially dys-functions. As most people, including myself, tend to have one or more symptoms in this area. I find it is a logical starting point to hear the wisdom within. Not every person is going to have a doctorate-level understanding of this topic, but fortunately one is not needed; just having an idea of how digestion works will help you unlock the code to a longer, healthier life. A great way to understand digestion is to think about it from a North to South process, starting with smelling and ending with elimination, with many processes occurring in between. In fact, just smelling or thinking about food can trigger the brain, which instructs our vital organs to release chemicals that start to break down foods. If we listen and tap into our wisdom within our gut will let us know if there is a breakdown in the system and what changes need to be made. If you focus on how you feel before, during, and after a meal, even for a day, you will begin to understand how this works.

Gut health begins in the nose and mouth. An immediate action item to improve digestion is to CHEW your food up to 20-30 times each bite. This will help to break down your food and absorb nutrients.

What we eat plays a critical role, not only in the quality of our life, but the length of it. There are fundamental questions you must ask yourself as you begin this process: "How nutrient-dense is the food I eat?" and "How does my body feel with these food choices?" As a simple beginning point, reduce the amount and frequency of consuming processed foods from a box, bag, can or drive-thru. As you do, next replace processed with fresh foods. Let this be an opportunity to find new recipes sure to delight your taste buds that deliver nutrients right to your system.

Once you have cleaned up your diet and are being honest about your food choices, you can then start to understand if there is a fundamental issue with your digestive system. If you struggle with food choice, I suggest you work with a professional who can help you with this process. I also highly recommend the Blue Zone lifestyle, which is based on healthy practices in "Blue Zone areas," or those with relatively high numbers of people living past the age of one hundred. These practices include living a purpose-driven and family-oriented lifestyle; it also means shifting away from the standard American diet, which causes inflammation and destructive processes through the body, including:

- Loss of barrier function. This results in leaky gut and, in time, your system will tag any food you eat as if it were a specific threat. If you find yourself eating food and feeling better only to experience symptoms again a few weeks later, know that this could be a contributing factor.

- Miscommunication of systems. If the system is always on hyperdrive and stress increases when the nervous system is supposed to turn on to digest, (which should occur while in a relaxed state), food will most likely just sit in the gut, causing symptoms such as bloating, gas, and indigestion. Long-term abuse of this system can cause significant changes in the appropriate digestive physiologic process.

- Infiltration of inflammatory cells into compartments where they are not normally found, which result in the overproduction of oxidants and cytokines. Once the system triggers constant states of inflammation and cytokine activity it is just a matter of time before the disease process occurs.

As the stomach, small intestine, and large intestine can all have this inflammatory response, a healthy diet plays a key role not only in disease prevention but in optimizing our energy, healing, and repair.

The next phase of digestion is the breakdown of our food. Once broken down the particles make their way into the small intestine, where absorption of vital nutrients and macronutrients take place. In *Molecular Biology of the Cell*, macronutrients are described as "proteins, lipids, and polysaccharides that make up most of the food we eat and must be broken down into smaller molecules before our cells can use them either as a source of energy or as building blocks for other molecules." When foods are not properly broken down because of gut dysfunction, the epithelial lining (cells that line the gut) will lose integrity and pathological conditions such as the passing of toxins, antigens, and bacteria into the bloodstream can occur. This can and will cause an immune response, further propagating the disease mechanism of the body.

Gut Check - do you experience bloating immediately following your meal? This can be an indicator that you don't have enough stomach acid. Yes, acid is essential for proper digestion. Get your stomach acid strong so you can break down the food and absorb nutrients.

Simple actions step, drink ½ ounce of apple cider vinegar before each meal. It is best to mix this with an ounce of water.

Cleaning up my gut, watching for food triggers, and giving my body the tools to heal were instrumental in my health journey. As you notice foods that disrupt your system, reduce how much and how often you eat them as a basic beginner's step to listening to the wisdom within your gut.

Stress also plays a huge role, both in our digestive function and our overall health. Cortisol, the stress hormone, causes inflammation in the gut, therefore stress management is essential to breaking the inflammatory cycle in the digestive system. Connecting with your wisdom within can help you recognize inflammation when it occurs and break this pathologic cycle so your body can heal.

The final stages of digestion are water absorption and elimination. This is where appropriate bacteria culture (known as flora) and other important organisms play an essential role, including that of histamine breakdown. Histamine is a chemical released by the immune system when the body encounters an allergen; is also found naturally in most of our foods. Breakdown of histamine is extremely important, as this chemical is critical for proper epigenetic expression of the DNA, it supports proper sleep wake cycles and can cause inflammation and chronic health issues like sinusitis, bloating, headaches, and even asthma attacks. When we understand this process, and that symptoms are helpful tools guiding us to make appropriate changes, we can start to become in tune with our unique system and, ultimately, rewrite our health future.

Gut check - if you have allergies or an inflammatory response, you may have a histamine imbalance.

Action step - stay hydrated, to find your ideal hydration amount, take your body weight in pounds and divide it in half. Now change that number to ounces and that is how much clean filtered water you should drink each day while also reducing foods high in histamines like: dairy, shellfish, avocado, alcohol, and processed or smoked meats. Note, this is a short list, there are many others that can trigger histamine responses in the body like tomatoes, beans and grains.

As you begin to listen to the wisdom within, remember, the first step is to own your health and start paying attention to and being present with your body, then choosing from a place of optimization instead of symptom prevention. In doing so, you will experience a higher level of energy and efficiency, our symptoms will "effortlessly" decrease or disappear, to live a healthier, happier, and longer life.

Dr. Amanda Krueger DC, FASA, ESMT has been owning and operating her own clinic since 2007 and been in practice for 15 years. She is currently finishing up her 300 hours in the DABCI program and will be eligible to sit for The Chiropractic B of Clinical Nutrition (CBCN) and The American Board of Chiropractic Internists (ABCI) next Spring. Dr. Krueger has spent her life continuing her education and getting to the root cause for patient's care. She recently finished her Nuerofeedback training and is a certified level II epigenetics coach from Apeiron. She has a fabulous husband and two wonderful children; two-year-old son and an eight-year-old daughter. Her passions include riding her horse with her daughter, competing in eventing, and living a life full of laughter and joy. Dr. Krueger is a strong Christian that focuses on biblical teachings and most importantly relationships.

https://whcwellness.com

CHAPTER SIXTEEN

The Role of Bioactive Nutrients in Longevity

Dr. Charlie Ware

The idea that what we eat and drink can dictate our long-term health and even lifespan is often overlooked by popular culture and modern medicine. As a doctor of acupuncture and epigenetic precision nutrition coach, my passion and path is working with clients from around the globe that are ready to enhance their health and life through the power of bioactive nutrients.

Most dietary regimens largely focus on weight loss and body image, with little consideration for the role our nutritional status plays in key physiological processes such as cognitive function and immune response, as well DNA methylation, which alters gene expression. Our nutritional status is dependent on the types of nutrients we ingest, and our body's current ability to receive those nutrients. A poor nutritional status, caused either by an unhealthy diet or by malabsorption of bioactive nutrients, is a major risk factor for many chronic diseases and early lowered lifespans. (Lola Corzo, 2020)

Studies show that bioactive nutrients are in part responsible for the evolution of humankind, bringing about not only certain phenotypic changes for example, the phytochemical folate acts as a methyl donor and is important for synthesis and regulation of DNA. A diet containing low folate content in pregnancy may have an affect on the future offspring and its health into adult-life, causing an obese phenotype and increasing the risk of hypertension (Sinclair et al., 2007).

Another interesting example, according to Dr. Stephen Cunnane of the University of Sherbrooke, directs attention to the upleveling of our brains and DNA. Dr. Cunnane points out that the brains of Neanderthals who lived along the shore and ate marine and sea plants evolved at a faster rate than the brains of those living on plains, away from water sources and subsisting on a diet of mammals and plants. He concluded that the shoreline diet, which was rich in bioactive nutrients exclusively found in marine life, allowed the Neanderthal's DNA to unleash a host of genes that affected the brain size of them and their progeny.

Dr. Cunnane is not alone in his thinking; there are tens of thousands of studies backing the claim that diets rich in seafood and sea vegetables not only enhances our nutritional status but have been linked to increases in epigenetic ages. The optimal diet is very individualized, and operates around a narrow range of nutrient-dense foods, lifestyle and continual self-governing.

Aging has long been believed to be a stochastic – or random – process, the result of changes in hemodynamics (blood flow) and the down regulation of organismal functions. Nutritional status, which can be measured by biochemical, metabolic testing and specific genetic markers, has a relational response to physiological processes used as markers to measure ageing, such as genomic instability, telomere attrition, epigenetic alterations, loss of proteo-stasis, deregulation of nutrient sensing/signaling, mito-chondrial dysfunction, cellular senescence, stem cell exhaustion, and alter-ation of intercellular communication (López-Otín C, Blasco MA, Partridge L, Serrano M, Kroemer G. The hallmarks of aging. Cell. 2013;153(6):1194–217.) The science of Nutrigenomics examines how our nutritional choices can slow or even reverse some of these processes to improve health, decrease the chance of disease, and give rise to the promise of longevity.

There are several organism and animal studies that bear this out. Bioactive nutrients were shown to modulate nutrient-sensing and signaling pathways, resulting in the activation of several cyto-protective processes including autophagy, antioxidant, proteo-static, and DNA repair responses. While most of these studies have demonstrated extended lifespans, on average, of between 10 and 19%, there have been a few where that number has been as high as 50%. Notably, pathways associated with longevity, such as insulin/insulin-like growth factor-signaling (IIS) and the mTOR signaling pathway, which plays a vital role in balancing anabolic/catabolic rates and regulating cell growth, were affected.

There are a variety of bioactive nutrients – terpenoids, carotenoids, essential oil components, phytosterols, polyphenols (flavonoids and non-flavonoids compounds), sulfur compounds, glucos-inolates and ally sulfinates, alkaloids, and polyamines, to name a few – whose role is to pass specific information between genes and pertinent bio-engineering processes. This bioinformation concerns the phenotypic expressions of the DNA that we can measure but also change with diet and lifestyle.

Our diet and, ultimately, our nutritional status, can help us achieve a life that spans well beyond the typical age. That said, there is nothing "typical" about our individualized genetic makeup, so our nutritional status should not be typical either. This is the hallmark of precision nutrition, which can give you access to the unique bioactive nutrients tailored to your genetic code. The best way to go about this is to have a Nutrigenomic coach map out a specific plan to you. The bioactive nutrients contained in the foods you are "prescribed" will help optimize your health and protect you from cardiovascular diseases, cancers, neurodegenerative diseases and age-related degenerative diseases. That said, there are a list of diets shown in clinical research to be bioactive nutrient-dense, antioxidant, and anti-inflammatory capable of modulating cell-signaling and key genes for phenolic expression and, more importantly, longevity.

The Ketogenic diet is a simple diet, meaning it is low in carbohydrates and high in healthy fats (mainly monounsaturated and polyunsaturated fats with some saturated fats). It involves dramatically reducing carbohydrate consumption in order to force the body to alter its metabolism to using fat molecules rather than carbohydrates as its primary energy source, and producing ketone bodies as a byproduct. In recent studies the keto diet has shown to activate many epigenetic factors, including the down regulation of inflammatory genes in the gut microbiome, thus reducing micro-inflammation. The shifting of the microbiome was achieved within five weeks and had a lasting effect even when transitioning to other less restrictive diets.

One great thing about the keto diet is the use of extra virgin olive oil (EVOO).

EVOO has been deemed the "nectar of the gods" in part because of its mentions in the Bible and many other historical records, but also because of its amount of bioactive nutrients, including several antioxidant characteristics that are of great importance to human health. While bioactive nutrients comprise only 1 to 5% of its makeup, the balance of mono- and poly-unsaturated fats affect the DNA in such a profound way that many experts, including me, recommend this as the primary oil to consume, for its anti-inflammatory, anti-cancer and antioxidant properties, as well as its modulation of glucose/lipid metabolism.

The Mediterranean diet has long been regarded as optimal because many studies have shown its ability to reduce lipid and DNA oxidation, ameliorate lipid profile and insulin-resistance, endothelial dysfunction, and inflammation. The protocol for this diet consists mainly of a high consumption of EVOO, vegetables, fruits, cereals, nuts, and legumes; a moderate intake of proteins from fish, meat, and dairy products, along with red wine; and a low intake of eggs and sweets. In addition to this ideal balance of proteins, low carbohydrates and fats, I believe one of the Mediterranean diet's many benefits comes from that region's use of herbs and spices, which have the highest concentration of bioactive nutrients.

For millennia, herbs and spices have been used, not only in cooking but medicine as well. There are thousands of well-researched and defined studies showing herbs as being curative, and complementary, with low toxicity. In the Mediterranean region, popular herbs include ginger, turmeric, basil and rosemary; these have been researched extensively for chemotherapy actions, antioxidant and anti-inflammation properties. They also have been shown to enter specific pathways in the body, promoting key epigenetic changes that pertain to health and longevity.

For example, caffeic acid, luteolin, resveratrol, gingerol, quercetin, curcumin, capsaicin, cinnamaldehyde and a host of others enter the Nrf2 pathways, an antioxidant pathway that helps stimulates the immune response to many pathogens. The Nf-kb pathway is stimulated when stressed. Without these nutrients, the outcome would be pro-inflammatory, however, these bioactive nutrients cause it to down regulate and not express inflammation.

Resveratrol and curumin are two of the most powerful SIRTUINS that impact the hallmarks of aging. Not enough due to dietary intake or a high stress lifestyle speed up the rate of metaflammation impairing cellular health, metabolic and immune function. Indeed, one of my biggest issues with the typical American diet, aside from the large quantities of saturated fats, sugars and simple carbohydrates, is the lack of herbs and spices to help with the inflammation ingested.

How do we obtain longevity?

- First individually we must define what longevity means to each of us. It is in my opinion that in order to obtain the precise nutrition for optimal genetic expression, one's specific nutritional profile has to be interpreted and honed to their unique bioactive nutrients. You may already have clues based on your heritage to consider traditional cultural foods as a beginning point with the next step being a genetic assessment for greater precision.

- Secondly, specific focus on the optimization of the absorption, the metabolizing and the detoxing of the bioactive nutrients is key. Breakdowns in these processes, as aforementioned, fail to be optimized in the traditional arc of ageing. Remember that incredible statistic, that some organisms fed their optimal genetic nutrients have lived up to 50% longer than their control counterparts.

  - Include bioactive phyto nutrients for enhanced absorption. An easy way to apply this is to eat a variety of fresh foods that are the color of the rainbow.

  - Metabolic optimization occurs when you decrease the amount of foods high on the glycemic index that break down quickly to sugar and spike insulin levels along with fried foods that increase cellular oxidative stress and inflammation.

  - Detoxing any toxins from the system can naturally be done by including herbs and spices into your daily diet such as ginger, turmeric, cilantro and garlic.

- Lastly, we must be aware of the constant changes in our environment that ultimately influences our resilience. We must be constantly vigilant in monitoring our biometrics in order to maintain our nutritional status to achieve our longevity goal.

The field of nutrigenomics is rapidly advancing. When you know your genetic blueprint, you hold the key to better understanding how to choose foods that are most optimal for you, making fad diets and one size fits all approaches to health a thing of the past.

Dr. Charlie Ware *is an international lecturer and researcher, renowned for developing products and wellness programs for several Fortune 500 companies. As the former Senior VP of BioLogics and a former Director to one of the leading health and beauty companies in America, he is a sought out natural health visionary. He is also the trusted US representative to the National Coalition for Good Governance of Nigeria.*

As a clinician, Dr. Ware specializes in Functional and Restorative medicine as well as Epigenetics and Genomics. And regularly works with CEO's, entertainers, Grammy award winning musicians, Oscar winners, NFL, NBA, MLB and other professional sports stars.

His passion can be best defined as "Developing concierge, precision, high performance programs designed to optimize performance." He has managed to distil complex and innovative concepts like epigenetics and genomics into bite sized, actionable pearls of wisdom. His method helps people take back control of their health and feel like themselves again.

www.drcharlieware.com

CHAPTER SEVENTEEN

Ancient Wisdom, Modern Practice
Learning from the Past to Design our Future

Dr. Ashley Beckman

Traditional Chinese medicine (TCM) dates back thousands of years and yet modern practitioners are still uncovering its secrets. For centuries, the ancient masters studied the healing properties of herbs and medicinal foods and developed many well-documented, effective practices that are backed up by modern theory. Moreover, many of the claims made in TCM can be validated with labs and scientific research, including those that explore cutting edge theories of epigenetic modulation. By utilizing the wisdom in the traditional texts, we are discovering how to alter our genetic destiny to live much longer lives.

TCM is not just about living longer, however, but about living healthier. Thanks to modern medicine and other factors, the number of individuals living to an advanced age is rapidly increasing. Unfortunately, chronic age-related diseases have also become more frequent. As a doctor of Chinese medicine and board-certified herbalist who focuses on healthy aging and longevity combined with epigenetics, my mission is to educate people on practical ways that they can adjust their lifestyle to avoid or heal these conditions.

For example, what we eat and drink can affect epigenetic changes (i.e. silencing or reactivating genes) that either significantly contribute to these diseases or slow or even reverse the aging process (Daniel & Tollefsbol, 2015). Martin et al. (2013) suggested that nutrition is one of the most critical external environmental factors because it modifies genetic expression at the transcriptional level. This is significant because the effects are long-lasting and extremely powerful. What you put in your body affects your epigenetic blueprint and has a direct impact on your health and anti-aging potential.

Regular use of specific, powerful Chinese herbs also holds the key to reversing aging and promoting longevity, as do other ancient practices. I believe wholeheartedly that the choices we make on a day to day basis determine how long we live and how long we remain vital and productive.

Epigenetics and Nutrigenomics

As mentioned above, aging is linked to the silencing or activation of particular genes. Epigenetics is the study of biological mechanisms that turn these genes on or off. Nutrigenomics is a facet of epigenetics that integrates genomic science with nutrition and other environmental factors such as cigarette smoking, alcohol consumption, and exercise. In other words, it measures how behaviors that are under our control influence our genetic expression.

The Epigenome

The epigenome consists of chemical compounds and proteins that attach to DNA, signaling genes to turn on or turn off. Once a gene has modified its function it is now "marked," which changes the DNA's instructions. These marks can be passed down from generation to generation, but they do not change the DNA sequence (Royston & Tollefsbol, 2015). While the epigenome can withstand many factors, it appears that modern-day living, including things like poor diet, lack of exercise, and smoking, is creating many malfunctions in the genetic expression (National Human Genome Research Institute, 2015).

Traditional Chinese Medicine

Published over two thousand years ago, *The Divine Farmer's Classic of Herbalism* is the oldest herbal text known in the world. This manual described in great detail 365 medicinal items and categorized them according to classes: superior food-grade tonics, medicinal herbs, and poisons. Related to the legend of the Divine Farmer is the saying that medicine and food are of the same origin. In TCM, this theory is still put into practice, through the creation of dishes that are infused with tonic herbs. These tonics are not used for medicinal purposes, but can be taken daily for longevity and radiant health.

TCM also recognizes an elite category of herbs, called "superior herbs," which have been found to promote longevity. Master herbalist Ron Teeguarden has said that, "The superior herbs provide this adaptive energy in abundance and are thus a primary source of true human empowerment." These precious herbs do not cure disease, but work with the body to "regulate the myriad of functions ... to remain youthful and radiantly healthy."

The principles of superior herbs are as follows:

- They help in lengthening lifespan. According to Teeguarden, "A tonic herb protects the body and provides it with a means to live out its genetic potential."

- The herb does not have side effects when used in moderate amounts.

- The herbs have the capability of balancing both emotional and physical symptoms.

- They taste good and are consumed as part of one's daily life.

Herbs such as ginseng, reishi, cordyceps, and green tea are some of the most potent superior herbs in Chinese medicine pharmacopeia that also have strong anti-aging effects.

Ginseng

One cannot talk about anti-aging and not mention ginseng. It is one of the most potent adaptogenic herbs and has a direct effect on the adrenal cortex, which is linked with the kidney system in Chinese medicine. The kidneys are crucial for promoting longevity through their gathering of jing, a precious energy related to the aging process. Ginseng has been widely studied for its antioxidant properties, which are the basis for their anti-aging benefits.

Longevity Tip: Take an herbal tincture or capsule daily; add ginseng powder or tincture to your morning smoothie or soup.

Reishi

Often called the "mushroom of immortality," reishi has been revered for centuries. The compounds work by protecting mitochondria and cellular DNA from oxidative damage. Reishi is considered to be the supreme protector – it affects the physical, spiritual, and emotional levels, making it useful for a variety of different conditions. It is also an immune modulator, meaning it will increase a lowered immune system and will decrease an overactive immune response in those with an auto-immune condition. Reishi spores are seventy times stronger than the mushroom itself and are considered to be one of the most potent immune modulators on Earth. They have powerful anti-aging properties, which is why they are considered to be an "elixir of life."

Longevity Tip: Take an herbal tincture or capsule daily; add reishi powder to your morning coffee, smoothie, or soup.

Cordyceps

Called the "caterpillar fungus" because of its elongated shape, cordyceps is one of the most treasured and expensive herbs, sometimes selling for up to $25,000 per pound! It has a unique ability to boost oxygen flow on a cellular level, protect mitochondria, and increase ATP, which increases energy production. Cordyceps is a powerful anti-aging tonic that can be used daily.

Longevity Tip: Take an herbal tincture or capsule daily; add cordyceps powder to your morning coffee.

Green Tea

Green tea is a Chinese herb that, while not prescribed in many formulas, is common in daily lifestyle recommendations. It is consumed daily on a habitual basis for therapeutic and ceremonial purposes. The chemical components of green tea, notably epigallocatechin-3-gallate (EGCG), the primary tea polyphenol, can protect people from epigenetic changes and help prevent specific diseases, especially diseases that are affected by environmental factors.

Tea is the most studied anti-cancer plant. Of the more than five thousand studies conducted on the medicinal benefits of tea in the last decade, over one thousand described its anti-cancer properties. The National Institutes of Health stands behind green tea as an emerging medicinal plant capable of influencing many types of cancer, cardiovascular disease, osteoporosis, and other neurological diseases (Uspenski, 2016). In human studies, the most significant results occurred when the consumption of green tea exceeded five cups or more per day. In vitro cell culture studies provided clear evidence that prolonged, high doses of green tea can change DNA methylation and reactivate genetic expression.

Green tea is also studied for its anti-aging properties, most notably with regard to telomere length and DNA damage reduction. One study (Daniels, 2010) consisted of 18 healthy volunteers who drank two cups of green tea daily for four weeks. The result was a 20% reduction in DNA damage. The telomeres of people who drank an average of two cups of green tea per day were about 4.6 kilobases longer than those who drank one quarter-cup per day, corresponding to approximately five additional years of life.

Longevity Tip: Consume five cups of green tea per day; add ¼ tsp matcha powder to hot water or smoothie daily.

Conclusion

According to vel Szic, Declerck, Vidakovic, and Vanden Berghe (2015), our environment is creating changes to our genetic code that makes us more susceptible to aging and disease. These expressions of change are included in the concept of epigenetics. As previously stated, epigenetics is defined as the study of heritable changes in genetic expression that do not change the DNA sequence, but change how the gene is expressed. Epigenetic expert Tollefsbol wrote, "What you do affects your genes. In other words, you're not predestined to a certain life because of your genetics, as we once thought. The genes you get from your mother and father aren't going to necessarily limit you for the rest of your life."

The evidence is clear. While modern scientists use different terminology, they have reached the same conclusion as the ancient practitioners of TCM: we can control our genetic destiny, and thus the power to create a long life filled with vitality and radiant health.

Dr. Ashley Beckman *is a Los Angeles-based doctor of Chinese Medicine, a board-certified Acupuncturist and Herbalist, and a certified epigenetic coach and functional medicine practitioner. Within her virtual practice, Dr. Ashley combines sophisticated functional medicine and epigenetic testing to discover the root causes of chronic conditions and creates a customized protocol for each patient based on their individual needs.*

During her last ten years as an acupuncturist, Dr. Ashley has performed over 45,000 treatments and also practiced with Dr. Soram Khalsa at the world-renowned Functional Medicine Clinic in Beverly Hills.

*Dr. Ashley holds doctorate and graduate degrees from Yo San University of Traditional Chinese Medicine and a degree in International Business and Marketing from the University of Texas. She is a contributor to the Huffington Post and Mind Body Green. To contact her or learn more about her work go to www.DrAshley.com or **drashley@drashley.com**.*

CHAPTER EIGHTEEN

Pain Resolution, Body Rejuvenation

Michael J. Meighen, MD

Pain Resolution: The Prescription for Longevity and Living a Limitless Life

Pain is an experience that is ubiquitous in the course of human existence. According to the Mayo Clinic, pain is the 2nd (Joint Disorders/Osteoarthritis), 3rd (Back Pain), and 9th (Migraines/Headaches) most common reason to present to a physician. Therefore, in total, pain is the most prevalent reason to seek treatment. The thought of pain and discomfort conjures up multiple unfavorable feelings which are detrimental to living a full and healthy life. Pain, however in my opinion, is an integral part of the health journey as it provides us feedback to the fact that we are out of balance and there is a compromise in homeostasis. The presence of pain is a multifactorial dysfunction which forces us to focus on comprehensive evaluation, rest, recovery, and restoration.

"A person who has their health has a thousand dreams, while the person that has lost their health has but one dream."

Two incidents in my life have served to outline this point and also forced me to examine options to maximize longevity, optimize health span, and pursue a truly limitless life. The first occurred at the age of 14 when I broke my right leg playing football. The injury was such that the growth plate was traumatized and caused a structural valgus irregularity in the extremity and laxity in the medial collateral ligament. I had two surgeries (one on each leg) to correct the deformity (right) and limit leg length discrepancies (left). The second battle involved coming face to face with professional burnout from my position as a physician. This negativity took a significant toll on my entire physical and mental being and ultimately destroyed my sense of self. Hope and joy were removed from my lexicon and replaced with anger and pessimism. While these stories are depressing and gut wrenching, they provided the impetus and fuel for exploration and embracing opportunities to heal. This pursuit has led me to an incredible tribe of healthcare innovators and disruptors that refuse to believe that the status quo is acceptable. The authors of this book including myself have created a revolution of thought and action on transformation for long-term vitality. Implementing the plan outlined in these pages will provide the template for all of us to live independently and at a robust level to the age of *One Hundred Fifty*. Yes, you read that correctly. *One Hundred Fifty*.

My name is Dr. Michael J. Meighen and I am board certified in physiatry (non-operative orthopedics) and pain medicine. I am a musculoskeletal expert and a health optimization specialist focused on total transformation of you, the client. My goal is to use all of the tools at my disposal, acquired over 20+ years of study and experience, to take you from ground zero to superhero. I use interventional regenerative medicine techniques including prolotherapy, PRP (platelet rich plasma) and mesenchymal stem cells to help improve conditions and dysfunctions related to orthopedics, aesthetics, and sexual health. I am the author of the #1 best-selling book on Amazon titled, *A New You: Using the Body's Regenerative and Restorative Healing Powers to Optimize Orthopedic, Hormonal, and Sexual Health Function.* I employ precision medicine techniques with a goal of resolving your pain points, fears, and limiting beliefs. This enhances the ability for you to evolve into a human "being" instead of a human "doing." I remove the barriers that restrict you and provide long term guidance for health span and continued progression.

These strategies have been incredibly beneficial in helping thousands of my clients achieve their goals by focusing on you as an individual or what we call an n=1 approach. In my estimation, pain management sucks as it serves to prolong the condition. My goal is to be the "Pain Disruptor" and totally revolutionize the treatment of musculoskeletal and pain disorders. The objective is pain resolution and functional restoration to enhance overall life span, health span, and well span.

The treatment and management of musculoskeletal pain in our country and worldwide primarily focuses on symptom management. The typical orthopedic surgeon, sports medicine physician, or pain management doctor will evaluate your specific complaint and focus their attention primarily on the area of discomfort. This myopic view will help a small percentage of the population, but typically provides only short-term, temporary relief as opposed to a long-term solution. The standard protocol involves a cursory examination, imaging (X-ray/CT Scan/MRI if approved by your insurance), high dose cortisone injections for the spine or joint (which have multiple deleterious effects on the body and longevity), anti-inflammatories and opioid pain relievers (which halt healing and decrease endogenous hormone levels), and surgeries. This cookie cutter approach allows the patient/client to fit into a 15- to 20-minute appointment slot, but consistently fails to address the root cause of the problem. Therefore, we have pain management which endorses continued interventions and drugs as a means of management. This style has the effect of disenfranchising the client and making them a passive participant in their care. In my opinion, this is counter to the goal of empowering the client and guiding them on a path to solving their issues.

My plans, therefore, are to cause a revolution and totally disrupt the manner that musculoskeletal pain is assessed, evaluated, and treated. My magic involves focusing on the client as a whole as opposed to a diagnosis. You are more than a knee or back problem. The issue is deeper than location and your pain on a 0-10 scale. We are all complex beings with multiple variables that play a role in our overall health. Thus, a precision medicine systems-based approach is the key for moving the client back towards homeostasis. In my opinion, the plan needs to be implemented in a proactive fashion instead of a reactive manner. Injuries will happen and acute management of these problems will still need to occur which I am well equipped to handle.

True health optimization and vitality comes from prevention as opposed to episodic treatment via the disease-based model (i.e. "Sick Care"). For example, orthopedic dogma on anterior cruciate ligament injuries of the knee was felt to be the result of acute trauma or a "one off" derangement. A recent study by James Ashton-Miller from the University of Michigan, however, placed this mechanism into question. He found that multiple inputs to the joint during training may cause microdamage and weakening of the ligament to the point where tearing may occur with submaximal impulse moments. Thus, this injury is more of a cumulative trauma and "lifetime achievement award" as opposed to an acute disorder. Moving forward, we thus may wish to treat college and professional athletes in the offseason with therapeutic stem cell ACL injections to reduce the incidence of injury during the season. This would have a dramatic impact on time spent on the disabled list/injured reserve list (as this is typically a 9- to 12-month recovery) and economics for the athlete, the teams, and the respective leagues. These non-surgical and medical options therefore would be perfect for companies and clients looking to reduce costs, maximize outcomes, and maintain the integrity of the anatomical structure while at the same time curtailing recovery time and boosting restoration.

Regenerative and restorative medicine started in the early 1950's via the work of Hemwall and Hackett as a means of treating joint laxity via the injection of sclerosing substances such as dextrose. The options for treatment include but are not limited to the skin, nerve, tendon, ligament, cartilage, bone, hair, and sexual organs.

Therefore, I am able to use dextrose, platelet rich plasma (PRP), and mesenchymal stem cells to trick your body into healing itself due to orthopedic, aesthetic, and sexual health dysfunctions. The beauty of these therapeutic entities lies in the fact that we are using the body's endogenous healing powers to create *A New You* (i.e. using you to heal you!). This reduces the risk for negative side effects including infection or rejection. The outcomes thus become more robust when you are optimized from a metabolic, hormonal, vitamin, mineral, epigenetic, macronutrient, and micronutrient standpoint. Enhancing these areas provide the necessary building blocks to heal and perform like *Wolverine* from Marvel X-Men fame. There are also a multitude of strategies available to elevate production of your own stem cells to further increase longevity and anti-aging effects.

Endogenous stem cell production is a necessary tool employed by the body for continued recovery, performance, restoration, and longevity. Optimizing and enhancing this measure requires a multitude of easy and cost-effective interventions that are available to the entire population. Ideal sleep patterns improve overall inflammation and reduce cortisol, promote anabolic repair and growth (primarily due to growth hormone, testosterone and progesterone), and enhance pain threshold. Optimal sleep is thus ultimately essential for the restoration of the body via stem cells. Exercise overall is beneficial for stem cell production in any form, but HIIT (High Intensity Interval Training), heavy weight resistance training, and Tai Chi are particular interventions with literature support. Hyperbaric oxygen therapy, infrared sauna, cold exposure, and pulsed electromagnetic field therapy all have positive effects on longevity and recovery. Caloric restriction, fasting, and intermittent fasting all increase hormesis and recovery via ramping up stem cells. These activities also increase autophagy encouraging destruction and removal of your dead and unhealthy cells (i.e. the body performs its own spring cleaning). Eating a cup of blueberries per day for at least 30 days significantly increases stem cell production. EGCG (epigallocatechin gallate) from green tea, blue green algae, and marine phytoplankton all are substances that positively increase stem cells. The peptide GHK-Cu injected subcutaneously also increases the production of stem cells.

I will now close the loop on the two issues I discussed in the aforementioned paragraphs which I believe looking back were milestones as opposed to problems. Life works in mysterious ways such that our lowest points may push us toward outstanding outcomes. Thus, discomfort in our past oftentimes provides the impetus for change and massive transformation. The musculo-skeletal injuries and surgeries that occupied my entire focus at ages 14 and 15 were truly a blessing in hindsight. This incident intro-duced me to the world of medicine, orthopedics, physical therapy, and recovery. It provided me with a pathway for a career and a conduit for focusing on my passion of precisely optimizing people. Dealing with burnout allowed me to take a step back and find out what was truly important in my life. Thus, I was able to reduce the clutter and drill down on things that were truly beneficial to my wellbeing. This allowed me to become a better human being. My goal moving forward is to write a book and host a summit on my experience to share with burnt out professionals. We all need to understand that we are not alone and that these issues may be overcome with help and direction. I want to give back and help to mentor my colleagues, thus reducing mental health issues, suicides, and career discontinuation.

I have now laid out a plan for maximizing your true potential for living a limitless and boundless life. My fellow authors will expound on other topics which will provide a complete pathway for you to totally dominate and crush it. In the aforementioned paragraphs, you have learned that simple interventions including sleep and nutrition are absolutely necessary as the foundation for optimal function and recovery. Once these principles have been mastered, then we are able to add the more comprehensive treatments including supplementation, bioidentical hormone re-placement, peptides, and regenerative medicine. The pearls of wisdom and take-home message from this chapter and the book as a whole is the focus on a systems-based approach to health as opposed to a disease-based one.

Data is essential for formulation of a plan to promote longevity, independence, and function. This sentiment runs counter to the current sick care model of health management prevalent in the United States where assumptions are made blindly without information. Third party payers in the insurance model are more focused on profits than health and thus restrict the acquisition of knowledge via denials. This reduces specificity and encourages a population-based trial and error approach which is more costly and less effective than the precision medicine model that we advocate.

Massive transformation requires massive change and implementation of the lessons in this book provide the essential elements for this evolution. The need to be proactive as opposed to reactive in all areas of your life become the mantra for longevity. You must become the solution and advocate for your own healthcare. Read. Review. Question. Implement. Now let's get out there and kick ass and take names together!

Carpe Diem!

Dr. Michael Meighen *Hi, I am a musculoskeletal expert and health optimization specialist focused on total transformation of my clients. I am the author of the #1 best-selling Amazon book titled, A New You; Using the Body's Regenerative and Restorative Powers to Optimize Orthopedic, Hormonal, and Sexual Health Function.*

I hold board certifications in Physical Medicine and Rehabilitation and Pain Medicine and have over 20 years of experience. My treatment plans primarily concentrate on conservative and non-operative measures to help the individual improve their function, pain control, mobility, and longevity. I use evidence-based interventions to restore, regenerate, and rejuvenate the client allowing them to live a truly limitless life. I employ proactive approaches including fitness and strength training, mindbody techniques, hormone optimization, regenerative interventional orthopedic medicine, peptides, epigenetic testing, sexual health interventions, and aesthetic procedures to maximize healthspan and vitality. I am confident that the client will progress and evolve if they are accountable and embrace the process. It is my professional opinion that the client must become comfortable with being uncomfortable and be willing to push the limits of precision medicine to become a super being.

My website is ***www.livelimitlessmd.com*** *and my email is* ***drmike@livelimitlessmd.com.***

CHAPTER NINETEEN

Inflammaging

How to Stop it and Reverse Age

George Rice, MD

Many of my clients ask how I got into precision medicine, a question for which there is no clear-cut answer. As with any endeavor, there were many interactions, experiences and people that guided me down that path. But the spark, that driving force that compelled me, was seeing one of the strongest people I know lose the strength to go on.

It happened on an otherwise ordinary day. I headed to the airport to pick up my wife, who was returning from a business trip – normally a happy occasion for both of us. This time was different. She was not smiling and it seemed to take every ounce of her will just to walk back to the car. The ride back home was emotional. She was spent. Done. She no longer had passion for her work. Physically, she could barely hold herself up in the seat. Her normally bright eyes were dulled. There was no energy in her words, thoughts or movement.

I felt numb. Scared. I had never seen her like this. Sure, she'd been sick before, but she was healthy, or at least without disease, now. So what was wrong? This set off a series of medical visits and specialist consults, who offered a variety of supplements, medications and procedures. Some things helped, some didn't, but none provided a permanent fix for her symptoms – fatigue, reflux, joint pains, muscle aches, difficulty sleeping, depressed mood, foggy brain and an inability to concentrate.

At that time, I had my own private practice, and like a good husband and physician I let others treat her while providing the support she needed. Though she received excellent care, however, there was no improvement; in fact, she continued to decline, which forced me off the sidelines and onto the field. I began to ask different questions that focused, not on what was wrong but what *wasn't right*. Why was she not able to make energy? What did she need for her gut to work well? Why was her immune system overactive and what did it need to return to homeostasis, or balance? This shift in thinking guided my own research and led me to a lot of other providers who were asking the same questions, and taking a systems-based approach to each individual rather than the one-size-fits-all paradigm typical of mainstream medicine. This was my first real introduction to the precision medicine movement, and it would not only help my wife but completely change the way I treat my own patients.

I began to apply some of the things I had learned about, starting with specialized testing, which in my wife's case revealed a significant hormone imbalance and gut dysfunction that the standard tests had missed. Finally, I had something to work with! Shortly after implementing some of the various tools used by practitioners of precision medicine my wife began to feel better. Her progress was slow but steady, and led to a long-term improvement rather than a temporary respite from her symptoms. Balancing one system led to improvement of other systems until she once again was the amazingly strong woman I had always known.

Seeing these incredible results inspired me to adopt this approach in my clinical practice. Addressing my patients' hormone imbalance made such an impact that I soon became known as "Dr. Feel Good." If you want to feel better and have sex, go see Dr. Rice!

This was just the beginning of my journey, however, because the more I learned, the more I kept asking myself, "What else don't I know?"

This quest, and my personal experiences, have led to my interests in cell function and how it plays out in our overall health. A lot of our health problems are driven by lifestyle, meaning the messages we send to our body from food, sleep, stress, and physical movement play a large role in the signals sent to our cells. Within the cell lies your genetic code and while your genes don't code for longevity specifically, they do code for secondary actions that contribute to aging. The cell rate of aging will slow down or speed up based on the quality of signals it receives.

Most people associate aging with those "inevitable" aches, pains, and a general slowing down that occurs when we accumulate a certain number of candles on the birthday cake. In the medical profession, aging is often understood and discussed in terms of accumulation of cellular and tissue damage that, over time, produces disease and ultimately death. Many signs point to chronic inflammation as the driver to cellular and tissue damage, called "inflammaging." Longevity, then, is the opposite, the avoidance of such damage; however, avoidance is not enough. We live in a time with access to science, information and resources that allow us to bolster the natural processes that repair cells and tissues that can slow down and even reverse the aging processes for enhanced health and function.

Yet, the biggest culprits sending in poor quality "signals" to the cells, speeding up breakdown and damage are stress, glucose and insulin. Each one signaling the next, this combo creates a negative feedback loop of sorts in the body that has a massive downstream and far reaching effect into every cell.

Too much insulin can be triggered from either high levels of stress or glucose. Ironically, stress produces glucose so the muscles can be fueled to "fight or flight" yet when you are not using the glucose, insulin is released by the pancreas to remove the glucose from the bloodstream back into storage. First into the muscles, then what is left over is stored as fat.

This chronic stress cycle is at play every day in the modern world often acting as a main contributor to weight gain or obesity. This produces a chronic inflammaging process from the accumulation of unnecessary fat in our tissues and cells. This metabolic process causes changes in fat cells that affects their metabolism and causes them to break down, which in turn triggers the release of inflammatory cytokines and activates macrophages. Macrophages are cells that kill bacteria and viruses; however, they also increase oxidative stress, an imbalance of antioxidants and free radicals in the body that are proinflammatory. The more chronic sources of inflammation, the more wide spread the aging process increasing the rate of breakdown and disease.

If inflammaging continues unmitigated, it then spreads to surrounding tissue and eventually becomes systemic, affecting tissue and organs far from the initial site – for example, liver inflammation can impair skeletal muscle performance. This "inflammation cascade" disrupts energy production, which then manifests as various symptoms depending on the organs involved, and results in diseases such as diabetes, heart disease and Alzheimer's dementia.

This chronic process where stress triggers glucose, which then triggers insulin, is aging you from the inside out.

Studies have demonstrated a direct correlation between obesity and advanced glycation end products or AGEs – a rather ironic acronym, given the topic. AGEs, which are fats that have combined with sugars through a process called glycation, are both made in the body and ingested through food consumption. Foods high in AGEs include things like red meat and cream cheese, however, they are often created during food preparation, as in the case of fried and processed foods. AGEs are markers of overall health – probably the best known example (and the first AGE to be discovered) is glycated hemoglobin, or "A1c," which is used to diagnose diabetes. They become a sticky like substance that interfere with several of the hallmarks of aging such as loss of proteostasis, and impaired nutrient sensing which trickle into cellular dysfunction.

Your body is able to handle low levels of AGEs, but if too many accumulate in tissues such as blood vessels, they can potentially cause significant harm. Tissue retention increases oxidative stress, which again can result in increased inflammation, impaired organ function and tissue death. Eventually, the whole body suffers the same fate.

Right now you might be thinking, if there is a way to activate inflammation, there must be a way to turn it off. If so, you are correct.

You can both turn off this overactive inflammaging and also bolster longevity from within your cells to look and feel your best for as long as possible. As mentioned before, while there are no genes that code for longevity, they do code for the secondary actions that can slow down or reverse the aging process.

This group of regulator genes are called SIRTUINS.

They are a family of proteins (seven in humans) that regulate cellular inflammation through sensing environmental and nutritional stressors. Sirtuins also play a central role in regulating metabolism, mitochondrial homeostasis, intracellular insulin resistance, and autophagy and apoptosis – two types of cell death that clear the body of damaged or diseased cells to make way for healthy ones. They both mitigate damage and enhance protection, which as mentioned earlier, is what we need to do in order to slow down and even reverse the effects of aging and age-related diseases.

Sirtuins reduce intracellular inflammation which is key to the age reversal process in several ways. They lower the activity of a protein complex (NFKB) that increases production of inflammatory cytokines; slow the activation of macrophages; decrease production of COX-2 (which promotes inflammation, fever, and pain); suppress inflammasomes (which activate innate immune response, increasing inflammation); and decrease the production of reactive oxygen species (ROS) in the mitochondria, which can lead to cell death and, ultimately, premature aging and various health conditions.

Chronic symptoms or decline in abilities are usually the first sign people notice that longevity is in decline. On an individual level, symptoms show up where there are genetic predispositions to imbalance or in areas that have been impacted by years of im-balance (e.g sleep deprivation, alcohol use, overtraining, joint overuse, et cetera). At this point, there has been enough free radical damage to mitochondria that energy production and therefore tissue health and cell function are significantly impacted. We complain of low energy, digestion problems, not sleeping well, weight gain, brain fog, decreased sex drive and motivation, and so on. We look for supplements, treatments, medications to address symptoms. The bottom line is there are a significant number of cells where mitochondrial function is suboptimal.

Many studies bear this out, including those involving type 2 diabetics which have shown lower numbers of mitochondria in muscle tissue, and that the mitochondria that are present make less energy. By lowering inflammation, sirtuins help maintain sen-sitivity to insulin, lessening the negative effects of excessively high levels of insulin. They also act to preserve a healthy number of functional mitochondria.

How Do We Address AGEs and Optimize Sirtuins?

- You are what you eat: Begin with what is on the end of your fork. Limit processed foods, restrict your calories (1,700-2,000 a day for women, 2,200-2,500 for men) and consume "Sirtfoods"which include: matcha green tea, extra virgin olive oil, kale, turmeric (cucumin is one of the most powerful sirtuins along with resveratrol), red wine, parsley, apples, blueberries and 85% or higher dark chocolate.

- Get lean: Through lowering visceral (belly) fat, you can enhance cellular function. A few tips to age in reverse as you get lean starts with daily exercise of 20-30 minutes moderate intensity to preserve lean muscle. Follow that with cold thermogenesis (think ice baths, cold showers and cryo-therapy) to activate the metabolically beneficial brown fat able to lower visceral white fat.

- Boost your cells: Another thing to do in order to optimize sirtuins is to increase your levels of Nicotinamide Adenine Dinucleotide (NAD+), which sirtuins need in order to function. NAD+ is a chemical compound present in every cell, and as our levels decrease with age we experience decreased cognitive and physical functions. Some ways we can increase NAD+ is through intermittent fasting, exercise, and consuming milk, certain types of fish, mushrooms, and green vegetables. We can also take supplements such as B3, that contain Nicotinamide Riboside, a molecule that aids the metabolization of NAD+.

To recap, any strategy to increase lifespan and healthspan must include minimizing cellular damage and maintaining the ability to repair damage that does occur; promote efficient energy pro-duction; and ensure optimal function of cells. Increased intra-cellular fat and insulin resistance lead to increased oxidative stress, which results in cells' decreased ability to detoxify and thus more susceptibility to damage, which we eventually experience as premature aging and disease.

We are constantly learning more about how to improve metabolic processes in order to prevent and even reverse this damage, and restore us to full health. What we do know is that minimizing AGEs and optimizing sirtuin activity, which allows us to avoid excess intracellular glucose and fat to prevent inflammation and insulin resistance, are the foundations for optimizing health and longevity. When you can reduce, slow down or stop the inflammaging process as shared in this chapter, you begin to add more quality years to your life, preventing disease, preserving and optimizing cell function, so you can look and feel younger for years to come.

Dr. George Rice *is known as an empowering guide to authentic next-level health. He is a specialist in Precision Wellness medicine. He believes that one should not just survive, but thrive. He is an expert clinician known for getting people to look and feel better than they thought they could.*

Dr. Rice combines state-of-the-art lifestyle assessment technology with cutting edge epigenetic coaching, peptide therapy, hormone optimization and functional medicine to guide motivated clients to their full health potential. He is passionate about helping clients develop the knowledge to attain next-level physical performance, a youthful appearance and longevity.

Dr. Rice received a B.S. in Psychology from Stanford University. He obtained an M.S. in Health Systems Management and an M.D. from Rush University. He completed his Family Medicine residency at the University of Southern California and is board certified in Family Medicine.

Dr. Rice is certified in Age Management Medicine and certified by the Academy for Preventive and Innovative Medicine in Advanced Bioidentical Hormone Replacement Therapy. He is certified in Functional Medicine through the Institute for Functional Medicine (IFM) and recognized as an IFM Certified Practitioner (IFMCP). He is specialty trained in Functional Medicine and Nutrition.

CHAPTER TWENTY

The Heart of Longevity

Dr. Gina Pritchard

Today, I know you CAN avoid a first or future heart attack or stroke. You CAN create the optimal health, cognitive performance, physical performance, and longevity you desire while achieving freedom from the threat of a cardiovascular event.

In the beginning of my career, I did not know this to be true. Traditional medicine taught us to identify, label, treat and manage symptoms, not correct underlying problems. There were no interventions taught at that time that would allow me to definitely tell you, you CAN live life without a cardiovascular event. After twenty-plus years of providing cardiovascular care in top-ranked hospitals, I experienced a sudden realization my practice had to change. I will never forget that day, and the look on the faces and in the eyes of that dear couple – both cardiovascular disease patients of mine – when their forty-year-old son was brought into the emergency room and pronounced dead from a cardiac event. Previously they had no knowledge that he too had cardiovascular disease, and witnessing their shock and devastating loss changed me forever. The truth is, I had seen that look way too many times in way too many people, but this was somehow different. I decided I could no longer practice as usual – providing crisis care and intervention when a disaster occurs.

I had to find out if anyone knew how to detect this awful disease early and intervene so that people did not experience what that family had. What I have learned, seen in my own practice, and know to be true is that crisis care for cardiovascular disease can be avoided in the majority of people. It is never too early and it is never too late to turn your health around and ensure you are protected. These greatest threats to the life you desire can be understood, and the potential for impact erased from your life.

If heart attack and stroke are optional, why are they still the number one killers and contributors to disability? In our current healthcare system, we offer the very best of cutting-edge treatment, medications, procedures, and technology to treat disease and save lives; however, our disease-focused approach does nothing to keep preventable diseases at bay.

The majority of heart attacks and strokes are ischemic – meaning the heart cells or brain cells are deprived of the oxygen and nourishment they need and eventually die. As mentioned earlier in this book, we are chronically over breathing, losing too much CO_2 from our system which impairs the exchange of O_2 and CO_2 at the cellular level. To reduce your risk, oxygenate your cells. Begin with soft, smooth, nose breathing at an ideal rate of 8-12 breath per minute.

Realize that a cardiovascular event does not begin in the heart and brain cells. Well before a heart attack or stroke and even dementia begins, the cells on the inside lining of our blood vessels, called arteries, become unhealthy and begin to show signs of disease; therefore, identifying, stabilizing, and reversing arterial disease begins with a careful look at the cellular level.

Science supports the fact that promoting health at the cellular level, and making precise recommendations based on one's individual genetic code, is powerfully effective. This is in agreement with the pillars of aging that involve genomic instability, epigenetic alterations, cellular senescence, altered intercellular communication, telomere attrition, and mitochondrial dysfunction. Before you decide this is all too complicated and think it may be difficult to fit into your life, let me assure you that understanding your areas of concern involves three simple steps: assess, adjust and live ageless.

Three Steps to the life and optimal health you desire:

Assess - What tests do you need? Learn about the simple tests (that you might not have had) that can make all the difference in your health and longevity.

- The Bale Doneen method allows for a complete genetic and blood serum testing package that will look at markers of inflammation, glucose, insulin, lipo protein, cholesterol particle size paired with genetic propensities.

- Check for arterial plaque. A coronary calcium scan, is a non-invasive, low-radiation imaging test, identifies calcified plaque buildup in the arteries of the heart.

- A blood test for C-reactive protein indicates inflammation.

- A blood test for the hormone NT-proBNP indicates stress on the heart.

- A blood test for high-sensitivity troponin T indicates damage to heart muscle. Troponin testing is regularly used by hospitals to diagnose heart attacks, but high-sensitivity troponin fine-tunes that measure, pointing to small amounts of damage that can be detected in individuals without any symptoms or warning signs.

Adjust - What changes do you need to make? Understand the small and large adjustments you can make in your life to achieve the physique, daily performance, and longevity you desire. This is best achieved in working with a coach or specialist that understands your cardiac data through a systems-based lens for total optimization.

Live Ageless - What does the ageless lifestyle look like for you? Simple monitoring, assessing and adjusting as needed. Get on with your life, enjoying the uninterrupted life of your dreams.

A comprehensive baseline assessment includes a look at the cellular health of your arterial system, inflammation, root causes and contributors, including genetics. The assessment is accomplished using ultrasound, computed tomography, blood, urine, saliva analysis, data-collection using wearable technology. In some cases, additional testing may be required. Once testing is complete, recommendations for adjustments to be made in your life are provided in the form of a ninety-day action plan with ongoing data monitoring and reassessments as needed, to be continued every ninety to one hundred twenty days after this implementation period is over. At this point you can focus on living your ageless life. Create your future story disease-free and dreams fulfilled.

Common questions:

1. If cardiovascular disease is still the #1 killer/disrupter of life, then what are we missing? Is there really anything else I can do?

    Yes – the first step, as mentioned, is to get a comprehensive assessment of your heart health.

2. Why do athletes and those who "live the cleanest lifestyle on the block" still have heart attacks or stroke?

    They were not given the opportunity to have a thorough look at inflammation and root causes. If you don't look inside, you don't know – even if you lead a healthy lifestyle.

3. Doesn't everybody have vascular disease – isn't it a normal process of aging? Can I really change this?

    Vascular disease, or atherosclerosis (plaque formation) is incredibly common but is NOT normal at any age. You can know where you stand with regard to healthy arteries and either maintain perfectly healthy arteries (at the cellular level) or stabilize and reverse any disease or unhealthy cells.

Remember, it is never too early or too late. Your future story can be different!

Gina Pritchard, DNP *is one of the nation's leading experts in the prevention of heart attack, stroke, type 2 diabetes and dementia. She is the owner of PREVENT! Clinic, located in the prestigious multidisciplinary institute, Model Wellness, in Dallas, Texas, and the Clinical Program Director for the Bale/Doneen Method. Dr. Pritchard's doctoral work focused on increasing global awareness and use of computed tomography and B-mode ultrasound for thorough, high quality assessment of the arterial wall, specifically the arterial intimal-media, to ensure arterial wellness. Her life work is focused on bringing life-saving, life-improving and easy-to-implement strategies to everyone so they can live out their long, vibrant, high performance, dream lives... uninterrupted.*

https://thepreventclinic.com

CHAPTER TWENTY-ONE

The Future Female: Hormonal Health

LaReesa Ferdinand, MD

Over my professional life I have had several heart-to-heart conversations with women of different backgrounds and lifestyles. Although voiced and articulated differently, they were asking similar questions.

The ideal is self-preservation. For example: "What can I do now that affords me the same level of independence as I get older?" or "How can I improve my quality of life today so I don't end up in a nursing home down the road?" Casually, women phrase questions based on avoidance of an undesired outcome; our conversations may focus on what we don't want, rather than what we truly desire.

There is no blame here; in fact, it is quite the opposite. Women are wired differently, and once we acknowledge that simple truth, we will stop comparing ourselves to men and embrace our own limitless power. That said, I want to be very clear on how we can create the life, and the health we want: *Start with the end in Mind, then Mind where you start to the end*. This piece of advice is founded on a quote from Albert Einstein, the understanding of which I have found essential to practicing the art of medicine: "We can't solve problems by using the same kind of thinking we used when we created them."

In my nearly two decades as an OB/GYN I have delivered countless babies, performed numerous surgeries, and helped women at all stages of life. I thank my patients for always challenging me and helping me recognize that my traditional training was not enough. I took the proverbial pulse of these women and realized that while our health is still defined by a diagnosis in one institutional setting, our conversations are being led by thoughts of healing our bodies "naturally." As the traditional medical curriculum was not fully marrying these worlds to make a bigger impact, they searched for answers on their own, only to learn that though we are in the Information Age, with an endless sea of knowledge at our finger-tips, not all resources are credible.

Seeking to fill this gap, I learned to curate my own path in the art of medicine through additional training in integrative, antiaging, and epigenetics tools. I like to use the word "whole-istic" because I have always viewed the Future Female as a complete package – composed of mind, body, spirit, and hormones.

Hormones are powerful messengers and mediators of vital func-tions of our body. They communicate with our target tissues and cells to regulate repair and growth. They are everywhere in our bloodstream and can impact everything. And everything can im-pact hormones. They set the stage in looking and feeling your best from your energy, skin, hair, mood, and muscle.

Women and men alike have the same powerful hormones with differing amounts most notably between testosterone and estrogen. While I specialize in working with women, the advice shared in this chapter also applies to men.

Environmental stimuli have the potential to impact our genetic expression, and thus hormones, which in turn changes our capacity to live and thrive at an exponential level. Hormones are the building blocks that integrate into your healthspan journey. The daily onslaught of stressors and endocrine disruptors leads to the mind and body becoming inflamed, right down to the cellular level. Advanced glycation end products (AGEs) are major hormone disruptors developed from exposure to chemicals and over processed foods that accumulate in our tissues and promote increased oxidative stress, aging, and hormone imbalance. The aging process decreases hormone activity and thus allows a part of the primary defense system to decline, making us all more susceptible to threats such as AGEs. This in turn, accelerates the appearance of aging in our skin, energy levels, muscular activity and ability to thrive. These inflammatory threats start as early as in the womb and postnatal period and are increased and decreased by everything we do. Over time, inflammation is linked to chronic disease and age-related effects. Hormone optimization is a key part of the equation. It's a fragile balance, but a necessary one.

There is power in the decisions we make every day, not only for ourselves but for generations to come. More and more research studies show that the way we treat our bodies is genetically passed down to our children and children's children, leaving them to deal with the effects. How we make these decisions all comes down to how we value our human experience and what we are willing to do proactively to lengthen our healthspan and lifespan, for ourselves and for our loved ones.

Future Female Longevity Power Tools

Power Tool #1: Start at First Base –The Brain

The brain is a safe haven for your thoughts, ideas, and aspirations, as well as vital biologic functions. Numerous growth factors, hormones and their specific receptors play a central role in the brain's function, as well as those of other organs and tissues. For example, estrogen, growth hormone, DHEA (dehydroepiandro-sterone), and testosterone are big contributors to movement of muscle and joint stability as well as cognitive function and memory preservation. Hormone levels also affect the brain's "plasticity," which is its ability to rewire itself and make new connections to learn, create new memories and skill sets, perform at a higher level, and delete other unnecessary programming.

As we age, these hormones decline, resulting in a decline in these functions as well. In my practice, I commonly hear, "Should I take hormone replacement?" and "I am on hormone replacement, but..." I am in favor of hormone replacement in the right scenario; however, it is not a one-size-fits-all approach. The real answer is to preserve youth at the most fundamental level: protect the brain and its inputs.

Various nutrient and hormonal cues function in the hypothalamus to control glucose and lipid metabolism and overall energy balance. Our energy sources are defined by responses to these and other conditions (i.e. stress factors) that threaten homeostasis, or the body's feeling of being in balance and "like home." When we make positive choices that create balance and reduce stress, we decrease the inflammatory cycle that impacts our brain's functions, thereby promoting the stronger neuronal connections that directly impact our state of being and purpose.

On the other hand, negativity, trauma, or the dimming of our internal flame creates inflammatory products that disrupt the very core of where our hormones and power stores work daily. This affects our weight setpoints, memory storage, metabolism, and athletic performance. It also affects our "WHY." When we allow our brain to work on our purpose, dreams, and visions, it epigenetically maps more calming emotions and behavior. Again, achieving balance depends on how we cope, react, make decisions, and internalize our environmental stressors and their impact in the brain.

Power Tool #2: Sleep is Queen

The antiaging and health and beauty markets are billion-dollar industries in which women comprise over 80% of the purchasing power. What most do not know is that the best anti-aging hormone optimization tool is free. I am talking about sleep, and even the priciest creams and serums pale in comparison to what it can do to restore us on the cellular and cognitive levels.

Let's think about what goes on during a typical day. Our brain processes millions of movements, thoughts, and patterns, most of them without our awareness. However, one of the greatest energy expenditures occurs during sleep. This is when the magic happens, the time when our cellular mitochondria, the powerhouses in our DNA, go to work orchestrating the repair and recovery productions. These repair mechanisms are controlled by the communication of our brain and body with our natural clocks, rhythms, and hormones. For women, this is critical. Disruptions can lead to a propensity toward obesity and metabolic disorders, and affect the extent to which we are able to express energy and harness our power to push through the next day.

As the science of epigenetics becomes more understood, the many truths it rests upon will emerge. The priority we place on maximizing sleep patterns with our natural biological clock, the better the return on our financial investment in health and beauty aids. Add to this the restorative powers of sleep with regard to cognitive abilities, and we see that the beauty it brings is not just skin deep. Prioritizing sleep is a powerful routine. This routine starts at the top of day, not when the lights go down. It's the intentional action in the morning to prioritize sleep at night.

Power Tool #3— A DNA Diet Births Limitless Willpower

There are two schools of thought around willpower (essentially you either believe it's limited or limitless), both of which garner merit. I believe willpower to make the right decisions fluctuates daily, depending on your food intake.

Our willpower often decreases apace with our work-life balance; therefore, the question of whether we can stave off cravings or indulgences should be explored on a deeper level. Have you ever considered, for example, that your gut is speaking to your subconscious brain, sending it secret signals that you need that which you crave? This is the biochemical reality, and one in which your hormones play a critical role.

An exploration of the gut-brain axis of communication provides a wealth of information on how our genes work for us. For example, when you eat for your genes it is much easier to exercise willpower. Your body's nutrient sensing pathways that serve as checks and balances help us make wiser choices toward cravings. These pathways become altered by the accumulation of insults over time and accelerate during aging. This creates more dysregulation of hormones for our metabolic needs and increases risk of obesity and inflammatory changes. A DNA-based diet mixed with intermittent fasting allows the opportunity to counter these changes with more renewable energy and willpower to maintain healthy weight and reduce the effects of chronic inflammation.

The Future Female Forecast

As you read through this book on longevity and the impact of epigenetics, you will find an underlying thread of nature versus nurture. Yes, we are born with a natural blueprint, but the choices we make, including hormone optimization, assist us in reversing the negative impact that chronic environmental stressors have on that blueprint. In effect, it wages cellular warfare on the elements that contribute to inflammation, skin aging and appearance, organ dysfunction and, finally, failure to thrive.

Each of us is tasked with finding out what choices we need to make in order to optimize our blueprint. Recently, I had a series of "a-ha moments," including the realization that, as a result of decisions I made years ago, I had moved away from my goals and dreams. I am not talking about my conscious decision to become a physician, but the subconscious creation of limited beliefs about my ability to impact women on a global level. Little by little, day by day, this limited mindset took away my power. My internal flame dimmed, and I experienced friction between my spirit and my life. You know what I am talking about; you have been there.

I realized that whenever you are not thinking and speaking in terms of limitless possibility, you beget less fruitful life experiences. Over a lifespan, this view of the future takes something away from you. It changes your perspective of yourself and the world around you. It keeps you up at night thinking about it. It impacts your willpower to make better choices the next day. This compounded stress creates loss of sleep and dictates the mood that drives your day. However, when we "mind where we want to finish" and uplevel our thinking accordingly, we discover our incredible power to not only solve our problems, but create the physical, mental and spiritual lives we deserve.

This is the Future Female mindset of health.

Dr. LaReesa Ferdinand *is a board-certified OB/GYN, women's hormone health expert, and the Chief Executive Wellness Coach/ Consultant of The Estrogen Doctor Company, LLC. She believes every woman deserves to live a healthy, beautiful life and age gracefully doing so. Her advanced anti-aging training, which includes hormone replacement protocols, metabolic and nutritional medicine, and epigenetics, helps women improve hormone balance to live more productive, powerful, and performance-driven lives through perimenopause and beyond. Her results-driven solutions are highly sought after in her business and speaking engagements.*

Dr LaReesa graduated summa cum laude from Xavier University of Louisiana; received her doctorate atLSU Health Sciences Center, and completed her Internship/Residency training at University of Florida Health Sciences Center-Shands Jacksonville. She has completed an Emerging Infectious Disease Laboratory Fellowship at the Centers of Disease Control and Prevention of Atlanta, Georgia, and is a former assistant professor and site director affiliated with University of Central Florida College of Medicine (UCFCOM). She was named one of the top OB/GYN Physicians of 2020 in the Orlando Family Magazine. In 2016, she was selected as the Most Outstanding OB/GYN Clerkship Physician Teacher awarded by UCFCOM.

She lives near Orlando, Florida. She is married with one child and enjoys relaxing with family, reading, traveling, and mentoring young women.

www.drlareesa.com

CHAPTER TWENTY-TWO

Peptides: Unlock the Secret to Longevity

Kent Holtorf, MD

Not a day goes by that I don't thank God for peptides. Peptides saved my life, and I have seen them do the same for so many of my patients, most of whom haven't seen improvement with standard therapies. I'm drawn to these complex cases largely because back in medical school, I *was* that patient. I suffered from terrible fatigue and was often barely able to function, only to be told by numerous specialists that my tests were normal and I was just depressed or stressed like every other medical student and needed more sleep or exercise.

I spent the next year investigating my condition on my own and eventually implemented multi-system therapies that resolved my most severe symptoms. Seeing these positive results firsthand changed the trajectory of my career. I left my residency and opened a center treating those suffering similar fates, and found my patients got dramatically better in two visits. I would go on to open twenty-two centers around the county and set up a franchise with an extensive physician training program.

Unfortunately, during this time of incredible professional growth, I was also going through a stressful divorce which resulted in a huge flare, leaving me mostly bedbound for months with debilitating fatigue, anxiety, panic attacks, a severe sleep disorder, profuse sweating, neuropathy, complete inability to handle stress, and allodynia (skin hurts with normal touch), along with many other symptoms. I then went into heart failure and intermittent AFib. I could not stand upright or walk upstairs, and I developed auto-immune kidney disease and antiphospholipid syndrome.

After extensive testing, I was diagnosed with Lyme disease, Babesia, and Bartonella (parasites that affect the red blood cells and blood vessels), along with a number of reactivated viruses and mold toxicity. I tried massive doses of intravenous antibiotics with no improvement, and no wonder – my immune system was barely functioning. My natural killer cell function ran between 0 and 3 LU (lytic units)—normal is > 30 LU. I remember being in the ICU with sepsis and overhearing the nurses outside my room say, "This is the AIDS patient that keeps coming up negative for HIV." Yet, the infectious disease doctors remained disinterested, and told me they didn't believe in chronic Lyme disease, CFS, or fibromyalgia and therefore would not address anything other than the acute infection.

I decided to go around the world in search of a therapy that could help me. Though I felt horrible, I had no choice – the infections were killing me. While many treatments I found were somewhat helpful, I still struggled to get out of bed every day and remained in heart failure.

The game-changer occurred while I was in Europe. I discovered and tried peptides, and immediately felt different. By the six-month mark, I was a different person. To the astonishment of my cardiologist, who had told me I might see 10% improvement in ten years, I returned to normal cardiac function in less than one year. He had never seen such a recovery. I also found a number of therapies that were very synergistic with the peptides.

What Are Peptides?

Like many seeking ways to improve their health, you've probably come across the term "peptides" and wondered what they are. A peptide is a compound made of two or more (but less than 50) amino acids (AAs) linked in a chain. (If this chain has more than 50 amino acids it is considered a protein.) You may also hear terms like oligopeptide (a peptide with less than twenty AAs); dipeptides (two AAs); tripeptides (three AAs); tetrapeptides (four AAs); and so on. A polypeptide is a long, continuous unbranched peptide chain.

Peptides regulate most every known process and system in the body, including hormone production, immune function, the sleep cycle, the production of inflammatory mediators, DNA replication, cell division and renewal, cancer cell destruction, libido, weight loss and lean muscle gain, mitochondrial function, cognitive function, mood, energy and other metabolic activities, tissue healing and specific biological functioning of the brain, skin, eyes, urinary and reproductive systems, aging and longevity, and many more.

When used therapeutically, they are much less likely to cause serious side effects than medications and hormones, in part because some are naturally occurring and degrading the body. In fact, many commonly used peptides have no side effects at all, even when given at doses 1000 times the usual dose, which is unheard of with any medication, or even water! They also have no known toxicity level, no matter how high the dose.

General Classes of Peptides

There are many ways to classify peptides, but the best way to fully understand how they can be utilized is to do so by location and main activity.

Immune Aging (Immunosenescence)

Immune aging is a known component of aging, contributing to the progressive inability to defend against infectious diseases, cancer, autoimmunity, inflammation, and cardiovascular and neurodegenerative diseases. A significant cause of immunosenescence is the progressive shrinkage of the thymus gland from about age ten until it functions at less than 10% in your 40s. Decreased thymus function disrupts the balance in the immune system among Th1, which fights intracellular infections; Treg, which enables self-tolerance, and Th2/Th17, which fights extracellular infections and induces inflammation and autoimmunity.

This disruption, or "Th1/Treg to Th2/Th17 shift," is exacerbated by any chronic illness (particularly cardiovascular, autoimmune disease and CFS), aging, stress, obesity, depression, anxiety, chronic infections, toxins, gastrointestinal (GI) dysfunction, and neuro-degenerative diseases, resulting in a vicious cycle of progressive illness and deterioration, rather than the normal repair and reju-venation. According to the US Center for Disease Control (CDC), approximately 80 % of aged individuals are afflicted with at least one chronic disease as a result of a declination of thymic related immune function.

Thymic function and Age

Knowing this, isn't it common sense to give back the missing thymic peptides that occur with age? That is precisely what integrative, functional, and precision medicine doctors are doing to reverse immunosenescence, with proven results.

There are several thymic peptides that reestablish a healthy Th1/Treg immune system, but they do have some differing effects. For example, Thymosin alpha-1 (TA1) is approved in over thirty countries for various infections and cancer therapy. In the US, it is FDA-approved as an orphan drug, meaning that like all of the injectable peptides discussed here it is only available at com-pounding pharmacies. In some cases, they are available as a supplement with strict manufacturing and regulatory require-ments.

Like TA1, thymosin beta 4 (TB4) increases Th1/Treg; it also reduces

Th2/Th17 and provides additional rejuvenating properties.

TB4 Active Fragment (Ac-SDKP) is a small part of the TB4 peptide that provides the majority of healing and immune-modulatory effects. It is only four AAs in length (out of the 43 amino acids present in full-length TB4), but is approximately ten times as potent per weight as the full-length TB4 and available as a supplement.

Thymulin, a bioidentical thymic peptide, is similar to TB4 peptide but has more anti-inflammatory effects than full-length TB4. When injected into mice starting at the age of 3.5 months, it resulted in a 28% increase in mean lifespan and a 2.8-fold decrease in the rate of cancer.

Body Protection Compound (BPC-157)

BPC-157, a naturally-occurring peptide in human gastric fluid, has numerous benefits, including the stimulation of capillary formation to deliver more oxygen and nutrients to tissues, as well as significant beneficial effects on leaky gut, the gut-brain axis, and the microbiome.

BPC-157 reduces inflammation and promotes healing in most tissues and systems in the body, including the gut; the brain (improves mood, cognitive function, traumatic brain injury); skin, muscle, and degenerative joints; the heart (prevents and treats arrhythmia, heart failure, and Lyme myocarditis); peripheral nerves (neuropathic pain); the bladder (incontinence); the immune system (inflammatory conditions, mast cell activation, and auto-immunity); is protective against neuro, myco (mold) and endo-toxins;, and improves insulin resistance; It is also antimicrobial, outperforming the antiviral acyclovir for the herpes class of viruses at 1/1000th the dose.

Gut-Brain Axis

There are two key aspects of the GI system that influence health and disease pathogenesis: the microbiome effects on the neurologic system, inflammation, and health, and the brain's determination of the microbiome through its influence on GI functioning. Essentially, if you have a leaky gut you have a leaky brain as well, meaning the blood-brain barrier (BBB) is not able to keep out toxins, infectious agents, and inflammatory molecules and cells. As mentioned, BPC-157 reduces gut inflammation and promotes healing of the gut, brain, and other tissues in the body; moreover, when combined with TB4 and TB4 Active Fragment, they form a powerful treatment with regard to the gut-brain-immune-inflammatory connection.

Pineal Peptides (Epitalon and Pinealon)

Epithalon, a four-AA peptide isolated from Pineal gland, restores impaired, aged, and damaged neurologic, immune, and the cardiovascular system, improves neuroendocrine and immune regulation, and prevents multiple age-related diseases, such as hypertension, memory loss, cancer, osteoarthritis, and overall mortality and morbidity in humans and animals.

Human cells grown in tissue cultures are only able to divide approximately 34 times, with the telomeres shortening with each replication, after which they age and die. This limit to cellular replication is known as the Hayflick Limit. Epitalon stimulates telomerase activity, which elongates cellular telomerase activity and allows cells to continue to divide and function.

Epithalon also slows down the aging of the reproductive system; increases thyroid hormone secretion; and improves glucose tolerance; it has also been shown to increase insulin production in old primates with insulin deficiency; and reverse reduced gene expression and protein synthesis in target tissues, as well as aging and illness associated with reduced mitochondrial energy production. Epitalon stimulates serotonin production and restores melatonin in elderly patients to the levels produced in young healthy patients.

Epithalon and Telomere Length (Hayflick Limit)

In a study of 79 patients aged 60-69 with severe coronary artery disease, half the group received six courses of epitalon over three years; they were then monitored for another ten years.

The functional age of the cardiovascular system of the epitalon group had progressed only seven years, compared to 16 years in the group that had not received it; they also had roughly half the cardiovascular mortality rate. Those treated with epitalon also normalized their circadian rhythm, increased melatonin production, and improved carbohydrate and lipid metabolism. Their physical endurance had improved by almost 10%, while the control group showed a significant reduction in endurance.

Another study investigated the synergistic nature of peptide treatment (specifically thymalin and epitalon) in 266 elderly patients over a 6- to 8-year period, resulting in improved indices of cardiovascular, endocrine, immune, and nervous systems, homeostasis, and metabolism. They also reduced rates of acute respiratory disease, ischemic heart disease, hypertension, osteoarthrosis, and osteoporosis, as compared to the controls.

Cerebrolysin

Cerebrolysin, a mixture of small molecular weight purified neuropeptides, is approved in many European and Asian countries as an intravenous injection for the treatment of stroke, dementia, and traumatic brain injury. A study concluded that Cerebrolysin treatment improved clinical symptoms of dementia – a 6.5-fold greater response than standard medical therapy available in the US – with few side effects.

Cerebrolysin is not approved for intravenous use in the US, but it is available orally as a supplement, which has been shown to also be effective in the prevention and treatment of the neurodegenerative changes seen with aging, as well as improving memory, mental performance, alertness, and concentration. It also stimulates new brain cell production, increases brain connections, and increases brain energy production.

Conclusion

Peptides are proving to be the ultimate anti-aging therapy, preventing and reversing the underlying causes of many aspects of aging and the subsequent decline in function and degeneration. This, along with their impressive safety profile, means they can potentially shift the medical paradigm from one of waiting to treat age-related diseases as they occur to one of prevention. I am a testimony to the power of peptides to reverse malfunctioning tissues, organs, and systems; I also see such effects on my patients, who were once written off by physicians as "untreatable." This chapter has only scratched the surface on the benefits of peptides, and I urge you to seek out more information and discuss your health and life goals with a practitioner knowledgeable in the use of peptide therapy.

Kent Holtorf, M.D. *is the medical director of the Holtorf Medical Group and the world (China and Thailand) and nation-wide Holtorf Medical Group Affiliate Centers. He is the founder and medical director of the non-profit National Academy of Hypothyroidism (NAH), which is dedicated to the dissemination of new evidence-based information to doctors and patients on the diagnosis and treatment of hypothyroidism and advanced integrative diagnostic and treatment protocols.*

He is also the founder of Integrative Peptides, which is dedicated to the training of physicians regarding ground-breaking peptide therapies for their patients, as well as bringing the highest quality natural bioidentical peptides as supplements with unique delivery systems to doctors. Dr. Holtorf is an internationally known lecturer, author, and innovator in cutting edge research and treatments.

https://holtorfmed.com

CHAPTER TWENTY-THREE

Longer Living with Technology

Dr. James Leonette

I'm a forty-one-year-old, out-of-shape former collegiate football player. I used to know what to do to get better, but I can't get out of this rut. My diet has gone downhill and I forget what it's like to have fun. I can't remember the last time I played. I'm stressed! Between all my kids' activities and work, I'm going downhill fast.

My heart is having issues. I was hospitalized for several days this year and don't feel like I've recovered yet. I'm scared of what will happen if I don't get back into shape and keep my heart healthy.

I want you to coach me back to health. My cardiologist recommended I get an Apple Watch for cardiac monitoring. I don't know what I'm looking at; I want you to review my cardiac signs regularly.

As I listened to my client's rather distressing monologue, my mind immediately went into assessment mode. I had a bit of a leg-up in this situation, as I had known this guy for twenty years; in fact, he had introduced me to my profession. As a friend, I had a vested interest in keeping him alive and well, but, I wondered, would he be worth sinking time and energy into as a coaching client? More importantly, would he follow my guidance and be a successful client? The more I thought about it, the more I realized he had already given away the answer.

Longevity is a cumulation of long life and high vitality, and many variables play into achieving it. In other words, if you want to know if what you are doing is working for you, don't guess – measure. Data is critical in almost every scenario. I have seven years of inspection experience, the majority of which was spent on medical devices. My purpose was to review records and verify data. I never hesitated to write up an organization if they failed to produce complete records such as software validations, equipment verifications, procedures, and production notes. Failure to document indicates breakdowns in the manufacturing process and, subsequently, adulterated products that don't live up to their life expectation. The same goes for us. The human system is far more complex than any device, and in order to optimize it we cannot rely on quick annual checkups. We need to get regular status updates.

The majority of my new patients do not understand their health data. Few have rudimentary knowledge of vitals beyond pulse and blood pressure. VO_{2max}, heart rate variability, oxygen saturation, and sleep patterns are all important biometric information that will allow you to detect anomalies that require further investigation. The goal of this chapter is for you to learn how to gather this information, and use it to improve your longevity.

As my friend's doctor suggested, the smart watch is the most practical tool for longevity assessments. No doubt you have seen someone taking a call from an Apple Watch or checking a text on their Samsung Watch, but their value goes far beyond these basic functions. Modern smart watches house an array of sensors that can give you instant health information.

Given the rapidly changing marketplace, it doesn't make sense to discuss any particular model of wearable device. It is far more important to select a device with sensors and software that have been fully validated with good clinical evidence to ensure that the data is accurate. Companies with published research studies transparently document the efficacy of their software and hardware.

Two developers that I follow are Firstbeat and HeartMath. Firstbeat made detailed connections between heart rate variability (HRV) and human physiology. HeartMath has a detailed heart-focused database and many clinical studies. Apple was the first to achieve FDA 510(k) clearance for a wearable ECG monitor. Passing that rigorous standard is a testament to how far wearable devices have progressed.

When selecting a device, there are several analytics that will provide the most benefit for your longevity goals.

Heart Rate Variability (HRV)

Your heart rate is constantly changing to meet the needs of life; the variation in rhythm provides a significant insight into your overall stress management and how your autonomic nervous system (ANS) is coordinating subconscious organ control. HRV, which is the variation in time between consecutive heartbeats, is a relatively new vital sign, having been discovered in 1965. Its clinical importance only became apparent in the 1980s, when HRV was confirmed to be a strong and independent predictor of mortality after a heart attack.

When it comes to HRV, a high variation is ideal. Think of the difference in blood flow required to reach distant tissues when you breathe, bend over, or are upside down in a roller coaster loop. Your heart and ANS need to constantly adapt to the stressors at hand, no matter how trivial. A higher HRV indicates an increased level of adaptability, which is an ideal situation for longevity. A lower score signals that your system is overwhelmed and not able to handle the current level of demand.

HRV has been tied to a variety of physiological functions that contribute to the score, including:

- Inhalation and exhalation

- Posture changes

- Hormones

- Metabolic processes

- Cognitive processes and mental load

- Stress, relaxation, and emotions

- Physical activity and exercise

It is important to recognize major impactors to HRV, including overall health, exercise load, medications, sleep, and alcohol. Multiple studies have demonstrated that short-term measures of HRV rapidly return to baseline after stressful events. Alcohol consumption generally reduces HRV for twenty-four hours, while moderate exercise will do so for just four to six hours. More powerful stressors, such as traumatic events, poor sleep, and working night shifts, have a greater impact and may ultimately affect your longevity goals.

One of the best methods to improve your HRV is HeartMath's Quick Coherence® Technique. This two-step process involves focusing your attention on the area of your heart while breathing slow and deep while making a sincere attempt to experience a positive emotion, such as a feeling of appreciation or care for someone in your life. A description of the technique is available at https://www.heartmath.com/quick-coherence-technique/.

Resting Heart Rate (RHR)

Resting heart rate is an ancient marker of health, with evidence dating back to 3000 BC. The importance of this biomarker is apparent, considering that humans and many other species average one billion heartbeats per life. There is a correlation between heart rate and the limits of basal oxygen consumption in life spans across mammals, amphibians, and unicellular organisms. From this, it has been theorized that a slower heart rate is indicative of longevity.

Your RHR should be between 50 and 60. For those with levels above 60, poor organ health may be playing a role. High blood pressure, higher body mass index, and reduced lung function contribute to elevated RHR. On the other hand, exercise, especially training within the moderate and vigorous zones of your heart rate (The US Centers for Disease Control have established these ranges as 64-77% and 77-93% of your maximum heart rate, which is calculated by subtracting your age from 220) will ultimately lead to a lower RHR. This is evidenced by highly trained athletes, who tend to have a lower RHR than the rest of us.

To reduce your RHR, it may be beneficial to first take an objective look at your level of physical activity, then make adjustments as needed. Increase your exercise load gradually until you start seeing your resting heart rate reduce. Look for trends over time, especially sleeping RHR.

VO$_{2max}$

VO$_2$max, which is a measure of cardiorespiratory fitness, specifically oxygen uptake, serves as one's baseline fitness level and is a strong and independent predictor of all-cause and disease-specific mortality.

Devices that assess VO$_2$max usually require at least ten minutes of sustained moderate running or biking to obtain a valid measurement. VO$_2$max values vary by age and gender – for middle-aged females, 35 or above is a good target; for males, it is 45 and up. Maintaining high VO$_2$max is critical for longevity. It is possible for a trained seventy-year-old to exhibit the biological age of an untrained fifty-year-old. Longevity optimizers should maintain large-muscle dynamic performance until age 60 to 70 (at a minimum).

Oxygen Saturation

Oxygen Saturation (SpO2%) is widely used for respiratory monitoring in critical care settings. By measuring absorption of red light (660 nm) and infrared light (940 nm) across a small area of skin, smart watches use a reflected light method that requires users to limit motion for accurate measurement. Given these limitations, SpO2% is primarily monitored during sleep and rest.

From a longevity perspective, SpO2% is an ideal tool in assessing cognitive function, exercise assessment, and sleep. Ideally, your SpO2% should be 95-100%; anything below 90% is considered low. Maintaining high levels is associated with enhanced cognitive function in elderly adults.

Attention to SpO2% should be incorporated into intense workouts. A drop in oxygen saturation indicates you have approached anaerobic threshold and are losing the longevity-promoting benefit of the workout. For frequent travelers, this metric provides insight into altitude acclimation and when it is safe to exert yourself in the new environment.

Regular aerobic exercise, breath training, iron-rich foods such as liver and green leafy vegetables are tools to help you improve your SpO2%. Mild hyperbaric chamber treatment increases oxygen saturation levels close to 100%.

Sleep

This is the most valuable information you will get from a wearable device. If you do not sleep well, your body cannot repair itself, cognitive performance declines, and HRV drops. If your device has a limited battery life, it is best to use it to monitor sleep than wear it throughout the day.

Wrist devices excel at detecting low SpO2% and sleep apnea, especially in the comfort of your own bed. Detecting and treating apnea is critical, as that alone will detract from every effort you make with regard to your longevity goals. Untreated apnea leads to high blood pressure, increased risk of heart attack, and loss of focus and concentration.

Measurement of sleep is complex. For simplicity, focus should be on sleep phases, RHR, and SpO_2%. Ideal sleep measurements are 50-60 RHR and >95% SpO_2%. Each device has its own language for characterizing phases. Generally, there is light, deep, REM, and awake. Target three hours of combined REM and deep, minimal awake time, and balance of light sleep. Seven to eight hours of total sleep time is needed each night.

Respiration

Normal adult respiration rate is 12 to 20 breaths per minute. A slower rate provides health benefits and many devices offer a slow breath training app. Physiologic improvement includes respiratory muscle activity, ventilation efficiency, sensitivity of cell biochemical receptors, HRV, and blood flow dynamics.

Exercise: Steps & Activity

Taking steps throughout the day does not, in and of itself, equal an active lifestyle. This means that a pedometer, which is a feature of almost every wrist device, only gives insight into how sedentary you are, rather than an estimate of your activity. Your ideal device will also measure a variety of activities and categorize each for aerobic and anaerobic benefit. In addition, multiple sensors will measure your stats while exercising, including heart rate, SpO2%, and respiration rate.

Garmin devices have an "intensity minutes" function that calculates the value of your training intensity and time. One hundred fifty minutes per week is the recommended starting load, though this depends largely on one's individual goals. I've recommended up to one thousand intensity minutes per week.

If you are using steps as an activity metric, be sure to calibrate your stride length to have an accurate distance traveled measurement.

Future Outlook

With the rapidly evolving market, we should see valuable improvements in wearable technology, especially with biosensors built into smart watches that monitor biochemicals such as glucose and lactate. We tend to associate the need for continuous glucose monitoring with diabetes, however, it provides valuable insight for everyone into how well they process certain foods and their effect on blood sugar. Lactate sensors provide key information on exercise intensity and monitoring the health of your heart, liver, and kidneys.

Conclusion

Taking the steps to live a long, healthy, and robust life requires a lot of inputs. Continuously measuring and monitoring your biometrics will give you and your longevity coach insight into how well your system handles interventions, from meditation and medication to diet and exercise. My hope is that you take this information and use it to begin understanding your physiology and interpret each input as having a positive or negative consequence to your longevity goals.

Dr. James Leonette *is an award-winning Chiropractor and Clinic Director of Enliven Wellness. He is native of Bridgeport, WV and graduate of Palmer College of Chiropractic in Davenport, Iowa. During the chiropractic program, he graduated with honors, served as President of Student Council and was a member of the Institutional Review Board that protected human subjects in clinic studies throughout the U.S.*

Prior to pursuing a career in health care, he served as an investigator with the U.S. Food and Drug Administration. He was responsible for inspecting medical device manufacturing facilities throughout Europe and Asia to ensure that they met the FDA Quality System Requirements.

Dr. Leonette holds a M.S. in Industrial Hygiene and B.S. in Medical Technology from West Virginia University. Dr. Leonette founded Enliven Occupational Health to assess and improve the health of workers at manufacturing facilities and extraction businesses. He is a Certified Medical Examiner (CME) and qualified to perform DOT driver medical exams.

Dr. Leonette holds certification by National Board of Chiropractic Examiners (NBCE) in chiropractic and physiotherapy. He is a member of WV Chiropractic Society and International Chiropractic Association. Dr. Leonette is a member of The Masters Circle and The Winners Circle chiropractic groups and regularly attends continuing education programs throughout the U.S. and abroad. Dr. Leonette has traveled to Dominican Republic with ChiroMission.

He is currently licensed as a chiropractic physician and/or acupuncturist in West Virginia, Virginia and Ohio. He regularly speaks to organizations about health improvement.

https://www.enlivenwv.com

SOUL

Follow Your Soul, It Knows the Way.

-Unknown

Through all of the research, beyond therapies, technology and treatments a common thread appeared again and again as a predictor of longevity ... that of wellbeing. The authors in this section invite you into the spaces and places calling to you from your soul that can enhance how well and how long you live.

CHAPTER TWENTY-FOUR

The Coherence of Gratitude

Dr. Jackie Kilraine

Let me ask you a question. If I told you there was something you could do that is proven to increase your lifespan, make you feel happier and more joyful, accomplish more with ease, boost your immunity, heighten all your senses, give you a great night's sleep, protect your brain from memory loss and it is so simple you could do it with your eyes closed, would you do it? Oh, and did I say it's FREE?

This tool is called the "coherence of gratitude," and in this chapter I am going to show you how to develop it using the power of your brain and heart. If you are like me, you like to know that this is proven and backed by science. Well, I have that covered. I will explain what gratitude is, how it rewires your brain, and how that affects your system as a whole. This includes optimizing your immune system, your physical brain health, and your cardio-vascular health, as well as increasing your lifespan. I will also explain how gratitude is scientifically proven to make your goals seemingly effortless to achieve.

I am the Director of Neurotechnologies for Aperion Zoh and the CEO of Expressing Optima, as well as a certified neurofeedback practitioner and epigenetic coach. I have been an examiner for the National Board of Chiropractic Examiners for over twenty years.

I am sought out for my Rediscovering You program, which helps women heal from past trauma and pain and go on to live their most fulfilling lives. I'm not just the doctor, though, I've gone through this transformation myself. After the death of my husband, I realized I didn't really know what was "just me" or what I really wanted. I had spent years giving away so many pieces of myself to others, and now I knew I had to reclaim MY dreams and desires to be a better mom, doctor and mate. This cultivation of brain and heart connection was a very big part of that process and it will have great benefits for you as well.

You start by beginning a practice of gratitude. What exactly is gratitude, you might ask? Merriam Webster defines gratitude as "the state of being grateful; thankfulness. Gratitude is a positive thought and positive thoughts lead to a state of well-being." Another dictionary notes that "Gratitude is advanced as a desirable human characteristic with the capacity for making life better for oneself and for others."

A 2003 study defined a grateful person as having four qualities. They exhibit a sense of abundance. They are appreciative of the contribution of others and their well-being. They appreciate simple pleasures. And, they acknowledge the importance of experiencing and expressing gratitude. Practicing gratitude is associated with an increased sense of well-being, which is shown to have mental and physical health benefits; it also plays a role in improving their interpersonal relationships.

Here's a fact that will help you better understand how this works. Everything begins with a thought. Cooking dinner, exercising, going to bed, making love, everything. You first think about whatever activity you intend to engage in, and in doing so you fire up the networks in your brain to create the action of that thought. What you are thinking and how you feel about those thoughts turn on specific areas of the brain. This leads to changes either positive or negative in your health.

This plays out in the research. For example, a study of a pro-fessional baseball team's group photograph was used to accurately predict the lifespan of the players. The players were all similar in age, were healthy and had fairly similar lifestyles. The study found that the bigger the smile of the player the longer they lived. A gratitude practice cultivates positive well-being which translates to experiencing more joy and happiness. In a review of the literature, Diener and Chan, concluded that the evidence clearly demonstrated that those with a positive subjective well-being lived longer and had less health problems than those with a depressed or pessimistic outlook.

Let's deconstruct what happens in the brain and body when we are grateful. Being grateful creates positive thoughts and emotions and this leads to an overall happier life.

Thoughts of gratitude induce a positive mood, which fires the left prefrontal cortex in the brain. This area is associated with positive emotions, secretion of the feel-good hormones, dopamine and serotonin, and helps to quiet the fear center in the brain. Negative thoughts, on the other hand, activate the right prefrontal cortex, which is associated with feelings of hypervigilance, anxiety and depression. An increase in the hormone cortisol results, which, in addition to anxiety and depression, also leads to weight gain, increased blood pressure and a shutdown of the calming parasympathetic nervous system.

Those with greater right prefrontal brain activation had a lower immune response, while those with a positive mood and higher right prefrontal cortex activation had a higher immune response. Numerous studies have recently shown that those with less subjective well-being and a more negative or depressed mood had shorter telomere length. Telomere length is considered a biomarker of aging.

Keeping the "use it or lose it" principle in mind, the more we have a certain thought or perform a certain action, the easier it will be to do the next time. This is neuroplasticity. The more often we feel and think positive or grateful thoughts, the easier it is to recreate that picture moving forward. A good analogy is taking a path through the woods. The one that is walked often is worn and clear. If you are not used to thinking positively, you will have to take a new path, trampling down the underbrush and clearing the saplings, but eventually the path will be easy to travel. The old path will become overgrown and less traveled.

Being grateful in even seemingly negative situations builds one's mental resources to deal with *all* situations. This has been termed "Broaden and Build" by author, professor and thought-leader Barbara Fredrickson. A gratitude practice broadens one's perspective, cultivating the ability to find the positive aspects of every setback, disappointment or failure; thus, laying the groundwork for us to flourish.

Other studies have focused on activating gratitude through the self-guided exercise of journaling. Those who developed a daily habit of journaling gratitude were found to have a more positive outlook and less health problems. They also exercised more and were more outgoing.

A nighttime practice of gratitude can also improve all aspects of sleep, from how long it takes to fall asleep to the quality and length of that sleep. Just fifteen minutes of gratitude prior to going to bed can cause these effects, though the results were directly related to how *deep* one's feelings of gratitude were. As getting enough good quality sleep can profoundly impact one's health, that is reason alone to begin a gratitude practice.

Coherence is a state of being when the brain and body come together through feelings and emotions aligned with the heart. It's a time when you feel your wholeness, the resonance that is you vs the busy doing of the mind and active state of the body each having their own agenda keeping you feeling pulled, disconnected and drained. Simply through noticing big and small, the moments you are thankful for, the surprises that are showing up, the moments that bring delight, each expression of gratitude aligns your mind, body and soul to express greater health, happiness and wellbeing.

So now we know through science that gratitude does the following things:

1. It creates a naturally calmer, more outgoing, more creative, more receptive and resilient brain, which in turn improves every aspect of our lives, including our relationships.

2. It makes us healthier and less likely to die of heart disease, diabetes and cancer. It increases immune function, and our brain's own immune system is more activated.

3. It improves sleep, which is critical to our overall health and well-being.

The facts are clear: gratitude has been proven to have numerous and profound benefits, physically, mentally and spiritually. And, when we make gratitude a practice, a meditation and a natural state of being, truly wondrous things begin to take place.

A meditation practice, in this case one that involves gratitude, does not need to be limited to what you can see and touch. Remember everything you do or say or create begins with a thought first. Your brain does not know the difference between what you vividly imagine and what is real. It will begin to lay down those neural connections, or clear the path if you will, the instant you create the thought. One such study that demonstrated this consisted of three groups. One group practiced playing a particular piece of music on the piano, another group imagined playing the same piano piece, and the third group did nothing. The group that actually played the piano showed an increase of activity in the area of the brain associated with learning music and, interestingly, so did the group that just vividly imagined or thought about practicing the piece! There was no change in the group that did nothing. In their study entitled, "From Mental Power to Muscle Power – Gaining Strength from Using the Mind," Ranganathan, et al demonstrated that simply visualizing performing finger strengthening exercises increased strength 35% after the twelve-week training period; moreover, when measured again four weeks later, after no additional mental exercise, the strength improvement was measured at 40%. Those who actually performed the exercise showed an improvement of 53%. There are numerous illustrations of musicians and athletes imaging future events to enhance performance.

A gratitude meditation practice increases our brain's production of gamma brainwaves. Gamma is a wonderous brainwave. It activates cytokines in the brain, which, according to a recent Georgia Tech and MIT study, can destroy the beta amyloid plaques in the brains of mice. These particles are associated with Alzheimer's disease. Human trials are currently underway using 40hz (Gamma) light and sound to activate this response. Gamma also heightens all your senses: sight, smell, sound, taste, and touch. It rides on the back of theta during sleep to all areas of your brain. Theta converts your short-term memory into long term memory, primarily during sleep (and we've already seen that gratitude enhances sleep). I look at theta as the magic carpet that gamma is riding upon. With gamma's sensory heightening ability, our memories are more vivid and more detailed.

Since we know every action begins with a thought and the brain immediately begins to build the "roads," if you will, to obtain the result of that thought, we should not leave our future desires out of our gratitude practice. Top athletes know this already. Michael Phelps has spoken about visualizing a particular swim every night before bed. When during the actual event his goggles filled with water and he could not see the wall of the pool, it was okay because his mind already knew where it was. He set a world record in that race. Other athletes, actors and others use this practice routinely. This practice, now understood with the science, helps us to prepare our brains and bodies for the future we want.

The best way I know to begin a gratitude practice is to allow yourself time in the morning to write what you are deeply grateful for. Don't rush through it; really feel the emotion as you speak to why you are grateful for this particular thing or future. This helps your brain build those neural pathways. I usually do this first thing in the morning and then again just before I go to bed. I may do more future pacing gratitude practice in the evening to give my theta and gamma brainwaves something to work on while I sleep.

I hope this has helped you understand how a gratitude practice will enhance your health and life. Enjoy! I wish you all the best on your journey.

Dr. Jackie Kilraine *is highly skilled at solving complex problems using a very individualized approach. This approach is designed to restore energy, remove fear, regain clarity and help clients look and feel ten years younger. Her specific approach utilizes advanced precision technologies such as QEEG guided neurofeedback and neurostimulation, precision based nutrition, sleep and supplementation as well as other advanced technologies.*

She is the Director of Neurotechnologies at Apeiron Zoh and the CEO of Expressing Optima. She is an examiner for the National Board of Chiropractic Examiners. She is the author of the Expressing Optima journal which is part of her Rediscovering You program. This program is designed for women to reclaim their joy and passion and to live life to the fullest to enhance their own life as well as the lives of those they love and serve. This path is now a system anyone can use. It is what is meant by Expressing Optima!

https://expressinghealth.com

CHAPTER TWENTY-FIVE

Foundations of Flow

Terry Clark

In a world where nobody really knows anything, you have the incredible freedom to continually reinvent yourself and forge new paths, no matter how strange. Embrace your weird self. There is no one right answer ... only better questions.

—Tim Ferriss

BANG! BANG! Flashbangs explode at 170 decibels and 40 milliseconds of blinding light.

"Police, Search Warrant, Open the Door."

No response.

The booming voice repeats the warning two more times, then the door flies open with the swing of the battering ram. We enter the room and in one cohesive unit sweep left and right as we flow in a practiced system of covering down threats from highest to lowest, careful never to sweep the muzzles of our weapons across each other's bodies. Our fingers off the triggers, we move smoothly and swiftly, rolling our weight from heel to toe with each measured step, ensuring we lift each footstep to avoid tripping or stumbling.

The above is day-in-the-life experience of a highly trained tactical team member executing a high-risk search warrant, be it in the clubhouse of an outlaw motorcycle gang or the home of a cartel leader or street gang member wanted for homicides and drug dealing.

How does one prepare for these tightly packed minutes, when they must operate at a high level of vigilance and yet not be overly amped or susceptible to outsized reactions to stimuli? The answer is a combination of foundational wellness and mental, physical, and emotional training.

While most "ordinary" people will never face these types of life-or-death situations, they do experience ongoing daily stressors that when not properly dealt with negatively affect the quality and the length of their lives. The question is, can we apply the same or similar approach as law enforcement to optimize our access to that type of "flow state"? As a precision wellness coach, I can tell you that the answer is an emphatic YES!

Each day, I bring to my coaching practice the experience and knowledge from decades in federal law enforcement and leadership study. I began this career in 1986, when I joined the Arapahoe County Sheriff's Office of Colorado after graduating college. As in most sheriff departments, that meant a job working in Detentions, directly supervising thirty-two inmates in the jail housing units. That experience led me to two epiphanies:

1. I would prefer investigating crimes and apprehending violent criminals over supervising them for eight hours a day, and

2. I needed to prepare physically, mentally, and emotionally if I wanted to survive and thrive on the streets while trying to apprehend violent young men.

Three years later that goal became a reality when at the age of twenty-six I was offered a position as a Special Agent in the Las Vegas field office for The Bureau of Alcohol, Tobacco, Firearms, and Explosives (ATF), the federal agency tasked with reducing gun violence, bombings, and arson. My duties covered all aspects of investigating these types of crimes, and in doing so my fellow agents and I often partnered with local, state, and other federal law enforcement agencies. There were times during my ten-year stint in Vegas when there were only four ATF agents responsible for all 1.5 million people in Southern Nevada, and it's safe to say we wouldn't have been able to get the job done without those other teammates.

Investigating these crimes always required the ability to run, fight, and shoot. The physical aspects were just a small piece of it, though; just as important were interviewing skills, knowledge of the law, complex problem-solving, creativity, empathy, compassion, emotional and social intelligence, writing and speaking skills. Two complex mental challenges were ever-present:

1. How to best acquire proof of the known suspect's criminal activity; and

2. How to identify the unknown suspect of crimes. (A "whodunnit")

As a member of the ATF Team IV Special Response Team, I worked to safely execute high-risk, tactical, search and arrest warrants, and participated in undercover takedowns, manhunts, and protective details on presidents, threatened witnesses, and officers. But I also conducted numerous suspect interviews, many lasting several hours, in which I had to continuously consider multiple priorities while maintaining engagement with the suspect. Specifically, I needed to:

- relate to the suspect to establish rapport
- apply the deep listening techniques of a therapist

- negotiate high-stakes outcomes

- use deception effectively when lawfully appropriate

- follow multiple layers of constitutional law

After a decade of first-line work I was promoted to supervising teams of agents, dealing with leaders of other law enforcement organizations and formulating policies and plans. Ultimately, I rose to Chief of Violent Crime Intelligence at ATF and was responsible for running data studies, analyzing patterns, trends, and anomalies, and formulating national solutions to reduce the gun violence rates in America's most challenged cities.

These experiences provided me with insight on dealing with stress from multiple sources. The most obvious is physical. The less obvious (unless you've worked in a vast bureaucracy) were the political, personnel-related, and particularly unsavory nature of working alongside ambitious career-builders who, after claiming to be willing to risk their lives for you on the street, would defame you, lie about you, or discriminate against you in order to promote their own agenda.

The latter of those challenges can raise your blood pressure, lower your HDL cholesterol, contribute to insulin resistance, disrupt your sleep, and increase your systemic inflammation – all of which can shorten your lifespan, depress you, and weaken your immune system. I know. It happened to me. It seems crazy that working in a federal office in Washington D.C. can be more stressful and dangerous to your health than arresting known killers in America's back alleys, but it is a fact.

All of us have faced challenges that increase the difficulty in accessing our highest cognitive performance, which is a necessity to experience the Flow state. We've also all experienced that feeling of Flow, individually and/or as a member of a high-performing team working as one organism. In every situation, our physical selves provide the foundation for the mental focus and emotional stability required to access the Flow state.

How can anyone develop the ability to survive and even thrive under immense stresses? Through a systemic approach to making lifestyle choices that not only build our resilience, expand our healthspan, wellspan, and lifespan, but also position us to access the Flow state much more readily.

In his 1990 book, *Flow: The Psychology of Optimal Experience,* positive psychologist Mihaly Csikszentmihalyi defined Flow as "...the state in which people are so involved in an activity that nothing else seems to matter."

Csikszentmihalyi also named the following eight characteristics of Flow:

1. Complete concentration on the task

2. Clarity of goals and reward in mind and immediate feedback

3. Transformation of time (speeding up/slowing down of time)

4. The experience is intrinsically rewarding

5. Effortlessness and ease

6. There is a balance between challenge and skills

7. Actions and awareness are merged so that one loses self-conscious rumination

8. There is a feeling of control over the task

You may have heard that humans use only ten percent of our brains, or that we need to use "more" of our brains to increase per-formance. These statements lack validity but tee up the discussion of Flow. Imaging shows that the Flow state involves the inhibition of the prefrontal lobe, which allows for more of the brain to communicate across regions. This enables one to make those non-obvious connections between disparate points – in other words, those "a-ha" moments of discovery.

Flow has also been referred to as self-actualization, or Eudaimonia. One study found that top executives were *five hundred percent* more productive when in Flow.

All of the aspects that contribute to your brain's ability to access Flow entail the elimination of limiting factors such as depression, anxiety, distractions, and "foggy" thinking, while simultaneously supporting calm, focus, and awareness. The optimally performing human brain relies on a body with lean mass, high VO2 max (maximum oxygen uptake), a high Heart Rate Variability (HRV), and the proper mix of neurochemistry.

Moreover, recent studies have shown that cognition and vascular brain flow work inversely to the degree of obesity. This fact reinforces all of the wellness principles described throughout this book. Here are the areas of lifestyle to focus on and tips to maximize cognition underpinning your ability to achieve Flow:

Sleep: Effective rest rejuvenates the brain nightly and sets you up for peak performance.

- Have a wind-down routine; avoid alcohol and caffeine too close to bedtime;

- Ensure your bedroom is dark, cold and quiet, with no clock faces or electronic screens;

- Get 8.5 hours of quality sleep per night;

- Wake within an hour of the same time daily; and

- Avoid checking your phone first thing upon waking.

Exercise:

Stimulates Brain-Derived Neurotrophic Factor (BDNF), an inducer of synaptic connections. Aim for sixty to ninety minutes a day.

Multimodal aspects are best:

- Stability work (foundational, i.e. Pilates)

- Strength

- Aerobic (Zone 2),

- High-Intensity Interval Training (Zone 5)

Nutrition:

- Selecting a diet consistent with your genome is critical;

- Match calories with body composition targets through intermittent fasting/time-restricted eating;

- Reduce/eliminate processed, baked goods, and fried foods typical of the Standard American Diet;

- Look for food sources with Carnosine (Beta-Alanine), Omega-3 fatty acids, Curcumin, Flavonoids, Vitamin D, Vitamin E, Choline, Vitamin C, Astaxanthin, Selenium, Copper, Iron (young women); and

- Limit saturated fat to less than ten percent

Breath: a daily practice of breath entrainment

Methods can be as simple as box breathing, observational breathing, pranayama breathing, or Wim Hof. All systems have value. Find the one that is suitable for you.

Mindfulness:

- Transcendental meditation

- Mantra meditation

- Movement meditation

- Focused meditation

- Spiritual meditation/prayer

- Mindfulness meditation

There are many mindfulness options available, individuals need to choose the one that works best for them.

Supplements:

Blood tests can confirm individual deficits of nutrients required to support brain function, including Carnosine (Beta-Alanine), Choline, Tryptophan, Tyrosine, Glucose, Vitamins B1, B3, B6, B12, C, D3+K2, E, Folic Acid, Pantothenic Acid, Zinc, Copper, and Selenium.

Once you have dialed in these other fundamental aspects, here are some higher-level options:

Brain entrainment:

- Neurofeedback (NFB)

- Transcranial Magnetic Stimulation (TMS)

- Brain Computer Interface (BCI)

- Hyperbaric Oxygen Therapy (HBOT)

- Floatation Tanks (REST) Reduced Environmental Stimulation Therapy

Nootropics:

- Caffeine
- Nicotine
- Lion's Mane mushroom
- Adderall
- Ritalin
- Modafinil
- Brahmi
- Winter Cherry (Ashwagandha)
- "Qualia Mind" a proprietary blend
- Ginkgo Biloba
- Maca root
- Yerba Mate
- Green Tea
- Aniracetam
- Phosphatidylserine

Plant Medicines & Psychedelics:

- Ketamine
- LSD
- Psilocybin
- Iboga
- MDMA

To be clear, I never used any plant medicines or psychedelics while I was a federal agent, as they were not legal. I am not advocating anyone violate any law or risk their brain by experimenting with nootropics or psychedelics without professional guidance.

The other aspects of enhancing cognitive performance I recommend heartily and use them in coaching my clients. The workbook I am sharing in association with this chapter will have much more detail on the specifics of the listed items and techniques under each heading.

We all experience episodes of increased stress that can diminish our ability to thrive, whether we are an agent chasing a serial murderer, a corporate attorney working in mergers and acquisitions, or a teacher facing a classroom of eight-year-olds. Increasing Flow is a worthy goal if you are seeking to improve your physical, mental, or spiritual wellbeing. Making lifestyle choices that contribute to improved cognitive performance will situate you for accessing and maintaining Flow so that you can make your desired impact on the world.

Terry Clark *FEDERAL AGENT TO EPIGENETIC PERFORMANCE COACHING: Terry's route to epigenetic performance & lifestyle coaching emerged from a lifetime of reaching for his own biological optimization. As a lifelong athlete he was tickled to refer to himself as a "professional athlete" because, as a Federal Agent for 24 years, he got four hours per week to work out. An insatiable curiosity and a passion for the hard sciences built a basis of knowledge that is very valuable in identifying patterns and trends and the significant anomaly in client's challenges in achieving their own best life.*

Terry understands first-hand how a stressful and taxing career can challenge your body and mind's ability to perform at its highest level. Identifying the links between a client's current lifestyle and impediments to optimization is just a first step in the epigenetic coaching model. Terry works with clients worldwide and resides in Maryland with his wife and son. He enjoys nature, CrossFit, rucking and studying all things related to performance, analytics and biohacking.

CHAPTER TWENTY-SIX

Love and Longevity

Dimitri Spanos

Contrary to what many of us believe, the length of our life has less to do with our genetics and more to do with the way we live – what we eat, how we sleep, socialize and practice spirituality, and, most importantly, the way we love. In fact, multiple studies have found that many incredible physical, mental and emotional benefits accompany the experience of love; they have also found that love actually lengthens our lifespan.

Love is who we are at the core of our being. It is an integral part of us and present within each one of our cells, just as we are an integral part of creation and woven into the very fabric of the Universe. As such, we are literally hardwired to know how to love one another; all we need to do is tap into our nature at a deeper level.

Love has no purpose but to fulfill itself. It lives in the desire, not in the attachment to any outside source. For any relationship to be wholly, deeply fulfilling and be able to evolve, love must be nourished and placed in its own sacred space, what I call the "garden of love." When we allow love to stand on its own and without attachment to the I (ego), love becomes an immensely powerful tool for living a long and healthy life.

We understand and experience the benefits of love through the heart. Our heart offers beauty and warmth and maintains all relationships between and within our cells, organs, brain, body, and the world. Our heart is also the center of all feelings—it is our joyful and loving compass of life and, if we allow it, will point the way toward health, happiness and abundance.

Discovering love and the higher capacity of the heart has been the topics of many books, workshops, contemplations and meditations. It has also been my longtime passion. For most of my life, I have focused on using my heart towards achieving greater love. It is the subject of *The Mind Is the Map*, which I co-authored, and my motivation for co-founding Eudaimonia Center, a learning center focused on achieving happiness for the highest human good. The Center offers transformational change, facilitating core healing and personal development. For the last ten years, I have worked towards developing strategies in Emotional Intelligence, using the consciousness of the heart and mind. As a practitioner of Heart Interiority and Alignment, I have been using methods of sustaining heart-consciousness as a way of living. Together, these tools provide a roadmap for using the intelligence of love to increase our lifespan and healthspan.

It is the processes of our mind that sends out impulses of Love and our DNA receives it. We are continually conversing with our DNA. Our emotions influence which genes are expressed and which ones are not. Every thought and emotion we experience sends a message which impacts each cell in our bodies and is registered in the memory of each cell. This cell memory imprints automatically and unconsciously and is later referred back to continually as this has our belief system.

It is our beliefs that alter our biology at every moment. When we are feeling unloved, isolated and tense our DNA contracts into tight coils. When we love and are feeling loved, our DNA expands into graceful spirals. In other words, it is our perceptions surrounding love along with our resulting beliefs that actually determine the expressions of our genes and our behavior.

It is our early experiences with caregivers that shape our core beliefs about love, about self, others, and life in general. Emotional experiences of love, nurturance and protection are encoded in the brain's limbic area, the emotional center. Over time, repeated encoded experiences become our internal working models – core beliefs about self-love, and love in relation to others, and love for life in general. These core beliefs become the lens through which we view our self, others and the world we live in.

When we understand that all the world is our community and all humanity is like family, we know that the concept of "Universal love" means that no one and no-thing is left out of the equation. This is the larger framework of love – when people come together, the world is a better place because of the love they share and generate. It therefore makes perfect sense that one's life expands when love, in any of its forms, is present. Our mental clarity improves, as does our relationships, both of which are likely to extend our life.

Dr. Waldinger is the current director of the Harvard Study of Adult Development, an ongoing analysis that has followed more than seven hundred men since 1938. More than sixty of the original participants, now in their nineties, are still taking part.

Over the years, researchers have interviewed the men in person, collected their health information (including brain scans and blood samples), and asked them to answer questions about their work and home lives, as well as mental and emotional wellness.

Those who are in healthy relationships have a longer life expectancy than those whose relationships are unsatisfying or toxic.

"People who are more lovingly connected to family, friends, and community are happier, healthier, and live longer than people who are less well connected," says Dr. Waldinger.

In addition, research from the HeartMath Institute shows that the experience of love, appreciation, care, and compassion leads to longer, healthier lives. Dr Rolling McCraty, the Institute's Director of Research, and his team have found that strong, loving relationships allow the heart to remain open and in "coherence," meaning our mind and emotions are in energetic alignment. Feeling heart-connected to others enhances our health and longevity.

Cultivating Love to Improve Longevity

Using a framework of self-love and self-care, we can focus on what changes we would like to make in our lives to prioritize our health. Shifting our perspective might include things such as working out or eating healthy as an act of self-love. These activities become less of a chore and they become much easier to sustain, in fact they can become enjoyable when we view them as an expression of self-love.

There are other healthy habits we might incorporate into our lifestyle that include all of those things we do which are good for us such as maintaining a balanced diet, exercise, allowing ourselves leisure time, getting enough sleep and meditation.

We can make choices more often which are kind and loving to ourselves. Ask yourself, "Is this the most kind and loving thing I can do for myself."

When we learn to love ourselves deeply, we have so much more love to share. Our relationships automatically improve because our choices stem from greater places of love, allowing for more frequent moments of happiness and connection.

Celebrate the moments which shape our lives and the support we receive. Our networks make the tough times easier to bear and the good times sweeter to savor. Connection, affirmation, community and belonging have all been proven to increase longevity.

While the heart's biological function is to pump blood through our bodies, it is also considered to be the physical place from which love stems and the place where love is received. In fact, it is the Heart which is the physical manifestation of love.

It is no coincidence to learn that so much of longevity, so much of life itself is tied to love. Our hearts keep us ticking so to speak, and when the heart stops, the body is left lifeless. We could say that life begins and ends with the heart, in more ways than one.

To summarize, science has shown that interconnected, intimate relationships provide people with happiness, warmth, a sense of well-being and wholeness, which in turn lead to a longer life. When we understand that we are love in action, and that love is literally embedded in every cell of our bodies, we start to respect and love ourselves. And love seeds within us greater appreciation for our blessings, compassion and empathy for those around us. One might even say that cultivating love, for the sake of love, both for self and for others, is the energy of life and the key to longevity!

Dimitri Spanos Co-Author of The Mind Is the Map and Co-Founder of Eudaimonia Center.

Dimitri was born in Athens, Greece, and has lived in New York for the past forty-five years. He is the co-author of The Mind Is the Map and co-founder of Eudaimonia Center, a learning center for offering transformational change, facilitating core healing and personal development, while empowering others to live extraordinary, healthy, and productive lives.

A successful entrepreneur for the past 30 years, Dimitri has developed concepts and tools for optimal performance by assisting others to identify their personal attributes and strengths and aspiring them to become Extraordinary Leaders in all areas of life. Dimitri Spanos, CEQP, is a Certified Six Seconds EQ Practitioner.

After successfully completing a three-year program and receiving certification in Heart Initiation, Dimitri has made a practice of working with Heart Interiority and Alignment, methods of sustaining heart-consciousness, a way of living his life. These combined skills come together to provide the expertise to write this book with such great passion, understanding the mysteries and mastery of the mind to live a more fulfilled and happy life.

CHAPTER TWENTY-SEVEN

The Soul of Connection

Jill Wright

I heard my father's harsh words saying "You will never make it in life" over and over in my head as I drove alone across the country to begin my new business. I had no idea what an adventure it would become. Those painful words inspired me to discover my purpose. My powerful desire for human connection was born!

At just twenty years old, I was the youngest person ever to be awarded an airport concession contract with The Metropolitan Washington Airports Authority. I was a determined young woman struggling to prove to myself and make my impact in the world. I would soon learn I was not alone, and this realization would change the trajectory of my life.

Though I was incredibly honored and excited by the opportunity I had been given, it also brought up all those tough questions around self-worth. I kept asking myself, "What do I have to offer, to people who are more highly educated and experienced in the world than I am?"

On the heels of this question was another, more expansive one: "How can I make a real impact and build a successful business?" The answer would not only become the foundation for Executive Shine, but lead me to a more satisfying and healthy life. The answer is human connection.

As I interacted with the vast cross-section of humanity that came for a shoe shine each day, I quickly learned that regardless of our ethnic, socioeconomic, religious or political differences, we all share the desire for real authentic connection. We all want to be seen, heard, honored and appreciated for our unique gifts. This was the secret sauce to happiness, and it was often found in the smallest, simplest of things.

One day, just for fun, I announced to my regular clients that I was going to have a contest: whoever wore the funniest socks would get a free shoeshine. The response was nothing short of overwhelming! "Oh my, what have I done?" I asked myself as I watched my professional, somewhat stuffy clients transform into competitive animals. I felt as if I had just opened all the cages at the Zoo!

I had just learned another powerful lesson. We are all just moving through life wearing different masks (and, as it turns out, different socks) with the one common desire to be truly 'seen' and acknowledged for who we really are.

For the past thirty-three years I have been privileged to witness the many mysteries behind those masks. This has inspired my lifelong fascination with discovering the genius that is hidden within all of us. In every environment there are unique opportunities to learn. My business has taught me "potential vision," to look beyond superficial appearances and reveal what's possible for everyone and everything. In a parallel metaphor, as we look beyond the dusty surface of a pair of shoes and see the "shine potential," we can look beyond the mask and focus on the potential within everyone. Regardless of their outer appearance or demeanor, we can acknowledge their inner beauty and help bring it to the surface.

Serving people by seeing people for who they really are, listening carefully and providing a safe place for them to belong is the foundation of our culture. I am honored that Executive Shine has been recognized by both Forbes and the Harvard Business Review for many of those "little" things that actually make enormous differences in people's lives, both in the moment and with regard to overall health and longevity. We have thrived and created longevity in our business as well, through a service model focused on authentic human connection.

Harvard has been researching the impact of quality relationships and human connection for eighty years, and their findings have been nothing short of incredible. "The surprising finding is that our relationships and how happy we are in our relationships has a powerful influence on our health," said Robert Waldinger, director of the study, a psychiatrist at Massachusetts General Hospital and a professor of psychiatry at Harvard Medical School. "Taking care of your body is important, but tending to your relationships is a form of self-care too. That, I think, is the revelation."

Our mission is to transform how we connect with people, both strangers and those near and dear to us. We begin by asking ourselves a few simple but powerful questions, for example, *What does love look like here?* You can replace the word love with many other words such as honor, compassion, kindness and respect – whichever you choose. By becoming present and asking these questions and then truly listening to the answers. You will have a profound impact on all of your relationships.

Some other foundational question includes: *What does love look like for me right now? How am I showing up for myself? Am I taking care of my needs so that I can show up as the best version of myself? Who am I being right now?*

Once you have met your own needs, things really get interesting, because now you can operate from a place of wholeness and satisfaction and you are then better equipped to make your desired impact and real connection.

Now, you ask that initial question again, this time with a different focus: *What does love look like for the person in front of me right now?* It doesn't matter whether it's a loved one or the person checking you out at the store – when you can take a moment to be present and ask yourself these simple questions, you shift from your head to your heart. You will also see a massive shift in your relationships and your quality of life.

With building relationships as my focus, I began to develop the art of human connection as a virtual treasure hunt. While being present and playfully asking fun, engaging questions, clues were revealed that led directly to the treasure within.

I also recognized that there is no connection in perfection. To build lasting connections, I had to set the tone by showing up as my most present, vulnerable, authentic self. For example, when I was vulnerable and asked good questions of my clients, I would watch them shift out of a stressful travel experience into the feeling of satisfaction that comes from sharing a positive memory. Something as simple as asking them to share their advice about where to take my mother for a memorable vacation worked to transform them right before my eyes.

Witnessing that shift taught me volumes about the power of questions and appreciation when building relationships. It reinforced my belief that all of us have the same basic need to belong, to feel valued, to be heard and understood. More importantly, we want to feel like we matter and are making a positive impact in the world.

I began to see my business as my secret way to bless others – to shift them out of their headspace into their heartspace. That single shift into presence, into true authentic connection, is the foundation of my sustained success to this day. It is one of life's greatest gifts to serve people and reflect their value back to them.

It's also the perfect covert love delivery system. If I hung a sign that said, "Love Available Here," no one would have the courage to stop by, but if I simply call it shoeshine, they line up all day long.

Our tagline is "Executive Shine: It's All About the Love," and it's based on the amazing power of human connection – a proven principle that has worked for over thirty years, and is the main ingredient of our trademarked Soul to Sole system.

Human connection has a direct correlation with how long – and how well – we live. As stated by Louis Cozolino, a professor of psychology at Pepperdine University, "Our brains are social organs, and that means we are wired to connect with each other and to interact in groups. A life that maximizes social interaction and human-to-human connection is good for the brain at every stage, particularly for the aging brain."

In his 2006 book *The Neuroscience of Human Relationships,* Cozolino cites the well-known, long-running Harvard Medical School Nurses' Health Study as one of the early indicators of how being socially integrated can lead to greater health, life satisfaction and longevity over time. Since then, the field of social neuroscience has expanded tremendously. In *Timeless: Nature's Formula for Health and Longevity,* published in 2018, he wrote, "People who lead extraordinarily long lives are those who have maintained close ties to others. Centenarians tend to be more extroverted and have higher morale, indicative of reaching out to others, giving and receiving support, and maintaining attachments."

There are many ways to live longer, better and more joyfully, but there is no way more effective or more natural than building authentic connections. Indeed, we are hardwired for it, and it is only our fears and limiting beliefs around our own value that stand in our way. I have found the best method to transcend those fears is by reaching out to others from a place of curiosity, compassion and, as I said, vulnerability. Yes, it may seem counterintuitive and uncomfortable at first, but once you see the results you will realize there is no other way to live.

Here are some action steps to help you experience even deeper levels of connection with yourself, in your relationships, within your community and the world.

Check in with yourself. Be more aware and conscious of your intentions. Get clear on your purpose. Ask yourself "What do I want and what are the steps to move forward today. How do you want to show up for yourself? Do something that feels good to you! Be responsible for meeting your own needs. You cannot pour into others from an empty cup.

Nurture your relationships. Think of it like caring for a garden. Sow seeds of kindness, listen, practice authentic curiosity and look for positive aspects to recognize. Remember what you focus on expands. Train yourself to look for the possibilities. Be patient and understand that people are just doing the best they can. Remember authenticity and vulnerability always own the room. People can feel your agenda so choose to speak from your heart and leave your ego behind. Science has proven that people can feel your energy before you even speak. So relax and share who you truly are and build an authentic connection, Soul to Sole™.

Build connections in your community too! Plan a potluck or barbeque in your neighborhood. Nothing brings people together like sharing food! Volunteer and support community organizations. You will meet like-minded people and become an important part of something greater! You have the power to change the world one connection at a time!

I invite you to create your legacy of positive human connection. Be present, breathe, laugh, listen, lead by example, engage in open authentic conversations, and connect with yourself and your community like never before! Be life-giving to yourself and to everyone you touch. Create a ripple effect of compassion that is felt around the world. Live your best life connected Soul-to-Soul with humanity, with nature and all of life, and you will see your positive impact reflected back at you.

Your long and joyful life may literally depend on it!

Jill Wright *is affectionately known as the Queen of Shine. She's a Heart Centered Leader and CEO of Executive Shine and has been recognized by both Forbes Magazine and Harvard Business Review for transforming the culture of client-based services. In addition, she founded The Shine Experience to share her 33 years of expertise, speaking and consulting to inspire leaders to unleash their human potential within their organizations through the power of love, honor and authentic connection. She is also a best-selling author and a host of the Shine Experience Podcast.*

CHAPTER TWENTY-EIGHT

Nature and Its Healing Power

Leann Spofford

"I go to nature to be soothed and healed, and to have my senses put in order."

— John Burroughs

Nature provides a place of comfort and solitude, an escape from the pressures of life. We yearn for the smell of forests and the salt water of the oceans. But does Mother Nature have the power to heal? More and more studies are bringing to light several truths: that nature has incredible healing properties; that we are literally hardwired to be outside; and that we have the ability, by becoming aligned with the natural rhythms of the Earth, to change the trajectory of our lives – mentally, physically and spiritually.

The question is, how do we harness this power? There are so many books, methods and modalities it seems we will never have time to absorb them all. And as we rush through our days in a frantic attempt to both level up and calm down, increase our happiness and decrease anxiety, we don't realize that we are passing keepers of great wisdom, and our key to a longer, healthier life. Those keepers of wisdom are the sights, sounds and smells of the natural world.

We are designed to be in vibrational frequency with the Earth. It is the devices and distractions of our modern world that throw us out of sync, leading and/or contributing to anxiety, sleep disturbances, a suppressed immune system, emotional imbalance and dis-ease. It is in reconnecting with the beauty of nature that we create our own prophecy, one of health, vitality and longevity.

As a Nature Epigenetics Coach, I help people realign themselves with incredible restorative powers of Mother Earth through nature immersion journeys and a discovery into the world of epigenetics. I came to this realization organically and quite by accident during my own healing journey. After a divorce and a challenging relationship, I instinctively knew I needed to spend time alone in nature. Each type of environment or part of nature has unique healing properties, and I've found that people are often called to one particular place or another for what they need in the moment. For me, it was the beach, soaking in the sun, feeling the salty air on my skin, and listening to the rhythmic crash of waves against the shore. While there I was drawn to a driftwood tree with unique grains, markings and limb breakage that I could only describe as "imperfect and yet beyond perfection." I named it the Beauty Tree, and the more I studied it, the more it brought me to a place not only of acceptance of, but gratitude for, my own perceived flaws. I came to understand that The Beauty Tree, and others like it are our teachers, sharing knowledge, holding space for us and showing us the truth of our own magnificence—emotional healing.

Most people recognize on some level that being outdoors is good for us. We remember those days from childhood, how good we felt after a day of playing outside; as adults, we know that a walk in the woods seems to magically lift our mood. For me, being on the beach produced an alchemical shift that had me wondering about the science behind it. What was it about being near water that made me feel so good? My research led me to the fascinating subject of negative ions. Negative ions are beneficial for the human body while positive ions (those from electronics) are harmful. Negative ions are abundant in nature, including moving water such as waterfalls and the ocean surf. Water in motion produces these negative ions, bringing us more energy and vitality. Studies have pinpointed several ways in which these ions contribute to overall well-being and health.

- They neutralize free radicals.

- They revitalize cell metabolism.

- They enhance immune function.

- They purify the blood.

- They balance the autonomic nervous system, promoting deep sleep and healthy digestion.

I also discovered several other scientifically proven healing properties of being on the beach that directly correlated to my increased sense of wellbeing. When I walked barefoot on the sand, I was activating several acupressure points in my feet and drawing in the charge of the Earth, grounding or Earthing. When I stared out at the vastness of ocean and sky, I was reaping the benefits of the color blue, which is proven to have a calming, meditative effect on the brain. Blue mind!

Water is considered the elixir and source of life. It covers more than 70% of the Earth's surface, makes up nearly 70% of our bodies, and constitutes over 70% of our heart and brains. That explains why floating in the ocean just plain feels good. I love being one with the ocean!

Studies illustrate the positive physiological changes that result when we spend time with trees. Aside from pumping oxygen to us, they release phytoncides, chemical substances that boost our immune system. Subjects of these studies have also exhibited lowered levels of cortisol, a stress hormone, as well as lower blood pressure and a decrease in pulse rate.

Being in nature results in increased heart rate variability (HRV), an indicator that corresponds with the quality and length of our lives. Going outside in the sunlight after waking up in the morning and watching the sky change from light to dark in the evening trigger biological processes involved with regulating sleep/wake times, energy levels and hormone production.

Nature immersion, which is what I facilitate with my clients, is based on the Japanese practice of Shinrin-yoku, or "forest bathing." This ancient healing technique is now being prescribed by practitioners in many countries. Shinrin-yoku is similar to meditation in that it is not about doing or forcing anything, but about allowing ourselves to move into resonance with the Earth.

What Does This Mean?

The earth is a living, breathing organism that vibrates at a frequency of 7.83 hertz. This is known as the Schumann Resonance, or what the yogis refer to as the sound of OM. This sacred sound takes the same shape as one of the most basic geometric forms in our universe, the ellipse. Sacred geometry, vibration & nature ... fascinating topics. When the human body resonates with that frequency, it goes into a natural state of healing. We are one.

One Sunday morning, in need of some grounding, I went snorkeling at Point of Rocks on Siesta Key Beach, Florida. The water was crystal clear, and as I glided along, enjoying the feel of the ripples of the water, I noticed the patterns on the sand below created by the sunlight. I intensely focused my gaze on them and was reminded of images of cellular structures I had seen. I felt as if I was swimming in neurons of the ocean, truly reaping the cellular healing properties of nature. It was a moment of profound realization of the power at our fingertips.

It is our natural state to be aligned with this power. When we are, we are happier and clearer in both mind and heart. Our immune systems are stronger, making us less susceptible to disease.

- In clinical studies, we have seen that two hours of nature sounds a day significantly reduce stress hormones up to 800% and activates 500 to 600 DNA segments known to be responsible for healing and repairing the body. –Joe Dispenza

- According to study conducted in Canada in 2015, "Having ten more trees in a city block, on average, improves health perception in ways comparable to an increase in annual personal income of $10,000 and moving to a neighborhood with $10,000 higher median income or being seven years younger."

- Researchers from Harvard T.H. Chan School of Public Health and Brigham and Women's Hospital found that women living in the greenest areas had a 12% lower death rate than women living in the least green areas.

- Soil contains a substance called mycobacterium vaccae, which has an effect on the brain similar to that of anti-depressants without any of the side effects.

Rediscovering and re-establishing this connection is much simpler than we may have thought. Researchers have established a threshold – 120 minutes per week – at which spending time in nature starts to be associated with good self-reported health and high self-reported well-being. Think of this prescription for "Ecotherapy" as the most effective one you will ever receive, bringing you increased joy, good health, and longevity. The first step is to regularly set aside time to unplug from technology that is causing interference and get outside. Schedule nature!

What do we do when we're there? Again, we do nothing. We simply allow. Studies have shown that we can experience nature through the five senses, each of which has its own healing properties. While walking or sitting in nature, take a deep breath and bring your focus to each of these senses, one at a time.

- Touch – Take off your shoes and socks and feel the grass, soil or sand against your feet. Touching animals have also been found to be calming; if you are in the presence of your pet or another friendly animal, slowly stroke its fur or feathers.

- Listen – For some, certain sounds, such as birdsong or ocean waves, are particularly healing. Close your eyes, inhale, and listen to the music of nature.

- Taste – Fix yourself a healthy meal made of things grown in the Earth. Eat slowly, savoring each bite of fruit or vegetable and picture the vitamins and minerals travelling to each cell of your body. Give thanks for the benefits the food has for your mind, body and spirit.

- Looking – Just gazing upon nature is calming and centering. Take a few moments each day to do so, whether it's a tree, a flower, the ocean. It may even be a picture of a forest.

- Smell – Companies have built an entire business model around the benefits of aromatherapy. But you don't have to purchase special scents; inhaling a freshly mowed lawn, a pile of sweet autumn leaves, or the rain will do wonders for your mood, and your overall well-being.

The good news is that society is beginning to catch up with science. Forest bathing, which is mentioned earlier has become a wellness staple in Japanese culture, is gaining prominence in other areas of the world; architects are designing future cities with nature and our inherent need to be close to it (also known as "biophilia"), as their focal point. In the meantime, if you live in an urban area and cannot completely immerse yourself in nature, there are still things you can do to soak it in. It just requires you to redirect your focus.

Cities bring a constant cacophony of honking horns, sirens, people talking and other noises that scatter our attention and energy and make it easy to forget that we share this space with nature. The next time you are walking around that concrete jungle, simply shift your focus from noisy manmade sounds to those of nature. What do you hear? Birds? Wind?

Most cities have parks or green spaces. Whenever possible take off your shoes and socks and stand on the earth. Breathe deeply and imagine the energies of the earth entering your bare feet and up through your whole body, infusing all your cells with love and light. If you cannot do this, reach out and touch a tree. Close your eyes and breathe. Can you feel the presence of the tree? Think about how long it has been there and what it has witnessed and endured, and how it has not only survived but thrived.

You can do the same.

It's your story.

Be limitless.

Escape into the healing powers of nature.

Leann Spofford *is a Nature Epigenetics Coach and founder of Nature's Beauty Heals – a wellness retreat to experience the beauty of nature immersion while learning how to harness the power of your DNA using epigenetics. Rebalance your life and connect to yourself and Earth on this nature immersive learning experience.*

Leann is also an experienced Marketing Director and Brand Expert in which she helps businesses remember and effectively communicate their "why." She is committed to helping people, businesses and nature prosper together.

Her upcoming book, Nature's Beauty Inspires, teaches us to draw on the beauty of nature and the power of gratitude to help us heal and create the lives we desire. Think Buddha and Louise Vuitton take a walk together in nature. She lives near an ocean in sunny Florida with her three teenage boys.

www.NaturesBeautyHeals.com

CHAPTER TWENTY-NINE

The Happy Formula

Matt Gersper

We all know what it means to "catch" a cold. Something from outside you gets inside you and makes you feel bad. When you catch a cold, your body experiences symptoms of that badness: runny nose, headache, cough, et cetera.

But what does it mean to "catch" your spirit? When something catches your spirit, something is triggered from inside you and makes you feel great. When *you* catch your spirit, your body experiences symptoms of that greatness: engagement, excitement, and enthusiasm.

Last night at 7:38, a text message from Melissa *caught my spirit.* Melissa is Dr. Melissa Petersen, the force behind this book and a dear friend with whom I instantly clicked the moment we met at a longevity event in the summer of 2019.

> *Hey friend, your [podcast] show layout is so perfect! Any chance that you would have enough time to write a 1,500-word chapter for the book, Codes of Longevity, in the next three weeks following a similar format to your show? Meaning [will you share] your formula and then break down your own story so that someone can understand and follow to express their own state of happiness? I just love all that you're doing and this is such an easy way to understand flow and format that I feel it could be a great read as well and possibly something accessible enough that we could get [your chapter added to the book] before the deadline hits for edits. Let me know your thoughts, no pressure.*

At 3:38 this morning, I replied:

> *I'm on it. I'll aim to have a final draft in your hands before the end of August.*

Now it's 4:53 a.m. and I've spent the last few hours tossing and turning and thinking about writing *this chapter*. Finally, too excited to sleep, I just start writing. Putting pen to paper as they say (or, more literally, thumb to keyboard on my iPhone).

And now, lying in bed, with my beautiful wife sound asleep next to me, I'm writing to you, dear reader, to explain the secret to happiness in 1,500 words or less. Easy peasy, huh?

The reason I haven't slept much on this night is actually also the secret to happiness ... it's what I call the *3 E's of Happy*: enthusiasm, excitement, and engagement. When I catch my spirit and I'm living there—in the 3 E's—life is inspired and flows easily. Writing a chapter for a book is a snap. "Work" becomes a joyful service because I'm operating from my true, unencumbered self. The real, authentic me, in-spirit ... the person I was meant to be.

The question is, how do we start living there? Here is the simple formula I've developed that helps me spend more and more time being happy, living in-spirit, and experiencing the beautiful symptoms of engagement, excitement, and enthusiasm.

Happy Formula: Capacity + Purpose = Happy

In other words, the "Happy" you want from life comes when you combine capacity with purpose!

Let's break down each of the three pieces, okay?

Living HAPPY

Happy, as I define it, contains four elements. They are:

> Doing things you love
>
> In places you love
>
> With people you love, AND
>
> Creating something of value to others

So, it's doing and it's giving... But to be a giver, you need *excess* capacity in your life.

Building CAPACITY

Happy is built upon a foundation of *capacity*.

I think of capacity as the ability to take care of myself and to have something left over to give to others. It's my personal responsibility to become fully optimized as a human being, utilizing the gifts that I've been given to create the life I want to live.

My capacity builders are physical fitness, mental fitness, financial fitness, and spiritual fitness.

Physical Fitness is all about strengthening the body, and encompasses not only exercise, nutrition, hydration, and sleep, but important health maintenance like doctor's visits, diagnostics, and bloodwork. It's important to note that the energy created by the practices of physical fitness are finite. What gets used up must be replaced with food, water, sleep, exercise, and so on.

Mental Fitness (commonly referred to as mental health) is all about strengthening the mind, and while not as tangible as physical fitness, it is just as vital. Mental fitness includes reading, meditation and reflection, goal-setting, creativity, lifelong learning, and the pursuit of hobbies. The energy created by the practices of mental fitness is also finite. The mind tires from use and must be rested, and its energy replenished.

I define *Financial Fitness* as building the financial resources needed to provide for yourself and others, and for me personally it is connected to a deep-seated sense of responsibility to do so. It creates the freedom to do the things I want to do and to enjoy them to the fullest, without financial worry. Of course, financial fitness is also finite. To maintain financial resources, every dollar spent must be replaced.

My philosophy of *Spiritual Fitness* is focused on discovering and cultivating the inner being that is my unique soul. Spirituality is learning to detect the differences between energy and ideas created by my mind (earthly energy) and those generated from deep within my awareness (spiritual energy). Spiritual Fitness is knowing that my inner spirit is my direct connection to the greater magnificence of everything in the Universe. It is my practice of holding and strengthening those moments when my "spirit is caught" and staying in-spirit more and more each day. It's awesome to exclaim that Spiritual Fitness is *infinite*. The more you use, the more you have. It's a lot like Love … well, actually, it *is* Love!

Before I move on to Purpose, let me share an amazing capacity-building concept called Kaizen. Kaizen is the Japanese idea that small, incremental improvements will add up over time to yield big results. As a personal practice, it means that there is always something I can do better tomorrow than I did today. It keeps me moving forward. Every single day. I may choose to work on a craft, or a physical skill, or a spiritual practice. I could be expanding my capacity for kindness, or becoming a better listener, or accepting others' perspectives more graciously. Kaizen can be applied to any capacity that I'm wanting to improve.

So, I've made it my lifelong practice to do whatever *I must* to build the capacity *I need* to take care of myself and my family and have something more to give to others. From that strong foundation, I do everything I can to discover and live my *purpose*.

Discovering PURPOSE

Happy is ignited by *purpose*.

In my second book, _Turning Inspiration into Action_, I explore the idea that major life transformations and "discovery of purpose" often comes from *devastation* – terrible illness, a sudden death, et cetera. That said, in the living of life I've found that a happier way of discovering my purpose is using *inspiration*.

I use adventure and love to discover my purpose.

Adventure helps take me away from the day-to-day. I relax my mind. Quiet my ego. When I'm thoroughly away and relaxed, that's when something catches my spirit and inspiration strikes. I pay attention to WHAT INSPIRES ME. Inspiration leads to my purpose and my purpose is where I want to live.

I define Love as doing things I love, with people I love, in places I love. One of the fastest ways to improve your happiness is to stop doing things or hanging out with people that make you feel bad ... a feeling that is the opposite of love. Recently, I've learned to even stop doing *good* things that make me feel *bad*. If I've taken up a new practice to build my capacity but I find that I don't like doing it, then I'll stop and find something else I can do to build up that particular capacity. So, I'd say, if you hate running, try hiking. If you hate meditating, try reading spiritual books. I am always trying to move towards Love because Love knows where my Happy is.

When I'm living in *my purpose*, I'm enthusiastic, excited, and engaged. When I'm in-spirit, my life is inspired, and it flows easily.

When you combine capacity and purpose, the sky's the limit. Can you imagine what it would be like to be doing work you love, with people you love, in places you love and creating something of real value to others? It's a very exciting life!

The magic of GIVING

That brings me back to the elements of "Happy," specifically, the fourth one, which is where I know the real MAGIC of life comes. Do you remember it? *Creating something of value to others.*

I knew that if I could do what Melissa asked of me—if I could break down my story, and share my Happy Formula so that someone (you!) could understand and follow it to express their own (yours) state of happiness—well, that would be *creating something of value to others.* And that got me feeling so engaged, and excited, and enthusiastic that I could hardly stand it. My writing was inspired and flowed easily.

At 12:49, this afternoon, I texted Melissa:

> *Guess what? I've just finished the first draft. 1,578 words. I'll reread and edit after lunch. Should have my submission to you before the end of the day.*

My friends, it is truly that simple. I leave you with a **HAPPY** challenge: begin a *lifelong* practice of paying attention when something catches your spirit, as if a *lifetime* of happiness depends on it. Begin it now, and never look back!

Oh, one more thing. I'd like to introduce you (to you). Please meet your true, unencumbered self. The real, authentic you, in-spirit ... the person you were meant to be.

I wish you a long, healthy, happy life.

With love,

Matt

Matt Gersper Mr. Happy Living

Hello ... my name is Matt Gersper, and I speak to people about finding true self. I have failed and I have succeeded. Lots of times ... Been hired. Been fired. Gone through a divorce and nearly drowned – separate occasions! Then one day at the bottom of a canyon, I woke up, took another chance. I found truth and joy. Love. Adventure. Significance. Things that matter most... to me! And now I live to give back. To help. To inspire. Books and talks. Retreats and Fun. I'm Matt Gersper ... Let's talk™.

https://happyliving.com

CHAPTER THIRTY

The Health of Your Wealth – Achieving Financial Longevity

Dr. Janice Hughes

Living longer, thriving lives is not a pipe dream. In fact, the very existence of this book demonstrates that it is quickly becoming our new reality. We have a new lens through which to view health and longevity, have set some new goals, and are taking actions that will enable us to live to one hundred and beyond. Yet it's not just about adding years to your life. When we think about longevity, a powerful and important question immediately springs to mind: will we have the finances and resources to live those years passionately and vibrantly?

I'm going to make a bold statement here, with a values-driven definition of wealth that I utilize with all of my clients:

True wealth is having the finances to do what you want, when you want, with whom you want, for as long as you want.

Notice I'm not just saying, "to have a nest egg," which may be construed as the need to live smart and be frugal with that nest egg. I'm not going to even cite the traditional financial planning advice or the six-step process to retirement. I'm not a trained financial planner; I'm a coach who helps people create a compelling vision for their future.

I've spent my life disrupting the traditional thinking around health and money, with an emphasis on helping people become aware of and focus on strategies that empower them to hold a very different vision for these aspects of life. This means putting yourself in the driver's seat and at the center of your plan, while utilizing experts and advisors to help you create and implement that plan.

This vision requires you to shift your DNA, take responsibility for your health, and take some of the vitalistic concepts about living vibrantly into discussions about money. One of the key things I found while in private practice was that as people age, they became more concerned about their legacy. This legacy included the health to do what they love and having the finances and cash flow to support those things. I was fortunate to attract into my own life both experiences and mentors that taught me about vitalistic approaches to money. This allowed me to begin teaching others these principles, and eventually use them to raise funding for a biotech company. It's these principles that I want to share here.

Money = Energy

Money is a resource, nothing more. Note that within the word currency is the word "current," which means flow or movement. It's like a river, or an electrical charge going down a wire.

Similarly, money has movement. It can circulate.

The energy can be converted from one form to another.

It can be blocked…yet it can also be opened up to flow more easily and effectively.

There is great power in understanding this. When we deal in currency, be it dollars, pebbles or some other form, we are exchanging it for a product or service. We are generating this currency from work we do, the things we create.

If money is just an energy, then how do we attract more? Notice I used the word "attract," rather than "earn" or "save." I am encouraging you to think of yourself as a magnet, attracting more resources and currency to you!

If I'm living to one hundred-plus years, I want to do things I love, with people I love. These connections with others are one of the most powerful aspects in all the existing "blue zones" in the world (those with the highest numbers of centenarians). Again, living longer and more vibrant lives brings up multiple questions for our generation:

- Why would I retire at age sixty-five?

- Do I have enough savings to live on?

- What reserves do I truly need to project and live to one hundred-twenty years old?

- What will my health and longevity care needs be?

The projections that have been used for the traditional financial planning models don't generally extend beyond age ninety. Statistics also reveal the lack of "retirement realists," meaning the people who have truly saved and created a long-term plan to have cash flow during their retirement years.

Part of the concept of living beyond one hundred includes the ability to purchase resources that help aid in our physical and mental longevity. To do this, we must build a new code – in essence, a new money "DNA" – that allows us to have plans in place to address the things that would typically have a negative effect on our financial well-being, including:

- What you think

- What longevity means to you

- Inflation

- What you eat (This falls under the "Rule of 219," which refers to the actual daily needs that are often ignored in retirement planning models)

- What you spend on healthcare and longevity care

- What you're paying to the taxman

These categories typically decrease your wealth and, ultimately, your freedom. Some we can control and some we can't; for example, it's not likely there's anything we can do individually to change inflation. The wisdom lies in knowing the difference, and in determining the simplest actions we can take to change or mitigate them.

Mindset Code

It's time to disrupt the traditional mindset that emphasizes that you "shrink your lifestyle" in retirement. In many cases that type of planning takes out your work travel, your spending for the family growth and career growth stages. This approach shows you how to conserve your capital and live on the interest. It also usually forgets to mention how many years you will be living, and living vibrantly.

Because Money = Energy, it's extremely important that we begin to talk and think differently about money and longevity. This means creating affirmations, or power statements, that set and establish a longer and more vital future, such as:

"I see myself thriving, active and involved with people and my community when I'm a hundred and ten."

"An abundance of reserves and cash flow allow me to travel, explore, and do all the things I love throughout my long and prosperous life."

"I am ... (fill in the blank)."

"I have … (fill in the blank)."

Thoughts become things! Write the new statements to build your new code, your new money and vitality DNA.

Strategy Code

Part of my mission is to help you be PREPARED, not scared!

You do this by learning vitalistic money factors, then cultivating savings and spending strategies that reflect that knowledge.

As mentioned earlier, disrupting the traditional mindset is key. Release the belief that you have to restrict your lifestyle once you retire, as many people do when they see their nest egg shrinking. Know that this belief is based in fear; it does not have to be your reality.

That said, we need to get really clear about our basic needs in retirement, projected out over a larger number of years so as to properly plan for our longer, vital lifespan. The Rule of 219 shows that oftentimes the amount of food we will need is not even considered in our retirement planning.

For most people, the primary residence is a major factor in financial planning, as it is probably their largest investment and the source of true equity. The question is, is it enough? If you were to access the equity from this asset while in retirement then what would happen to this asset when anything happens to you or your spouse? In essence there would be no equity left. In addition, many homeowners plan to pass down this property to their children or grandchildren, but to do this means they can't leverage all the cash flow from it.

And if we are to sell the "big home" to scale down, what portion of those assets would it take to truly have your basic shelter needs met? For example, in many cases the condo or retirement facility costs more than you have projected.

Action Code

What action can you take *now* to learn these vitalistic approaches? In other words, what can you do to become that "point person" in your own planning and strategies?

The first step is to write out the health goals and actions laid out in this book, as they will set you on the course to living, with vitality, to age one hundred and beyond. Then you can move on to establishing some actions around money.

Traditionally, our approach, both individually and through advisors, has been product driven. My focus, however, is on the process – what is the new thinking, planning, and strategies needed to create a new vision for your long and vital life?

One of my favorite tools is The 52-Week Money Challenge. In fact, I've watched my sons' "money DNA" grow based on learning and understanding the habit of saving, and what building reserves can 'feel' like. You start by saving $1 in Week 1; $2 in Week 2; and so on, until you save $52 in Week 52. At the one-year mark, you will have saved $1378.

This is a simple and straightforward way to help anyone learn the power and energy of a stack of cash. I utilized this exercise with my youngest son, who was an athlete and had no time to fit a job into his schedule during high school. He's now more "liquid" with his savings than most adults and married couples. He's become a "World Class Saver."

You might also check out *Inspired Wealth,* an e-book I co-authored a few years ago. It is chock full of information about the movement and energy of money. You can download it FREE right here: https://www.codesoflongevity.com/gifts

There are many other free resources that take a values-driven approach to money. Part of your action code will be finding these resources and incorporating them into daily life, as well as your plans for the future. Here's to your long and prosperous life!

Dr. Janice Hughes *is an Executive Coach and Business Advisor with one of the most impressive track records in the healthcare arena. She has worked with thousands of doctors from all walks of life, helping them overcome personal and professional challenges to reach greater levels of success. Janice's blend of intuition, practicality and incredible focus has made her a role model for professional women. It is those same skill-sets which she has translated into her key role as the Director of Investments for Curemark LLC. Curemark is a start-up biotechnology company which has matured into a major force in the area of autism and other neurological disorders where there is an unmet healthcare need. And along the way increase the value of the company from 20 Million to a valuation of over 150 Billion.*

Janice brings to her work a sense of urgency and intensity. Throughout her career she has worked in environments where convention meets unconvention, at the crossroads where health, science, and humanity all meet. This has allowed her to break through many barriers, both real and imagined. Her work underscores her life in that anything is possible, no is just a two-letter word, and with good leadership and a great idea one can change the world. Janice is committed to helping others create financial vitality to ensure they live long and prosperous lives! To learn more about her work reach out to drjanice@2inspirewomen.com and:

https://www.drjanicehughes.com

CHAPTER THIRTY-ONE

Spiritual Epigenetics

Giselle Koy

Longevity Codes. Divine Codes.

Longevity, taken to its full expression, is also known as immortality. It is mentioned in ancient spiritual texts and referred to as a form of the "holy grail" of human skills.

The Essenes referred to a time when they would regenerate their bodies to extend their lifespans in order to be of greater service for longer periods of time. They would withdraw from life and take sepulcher baths, after which they could live another hundred years or so.

In this chapter, let's lean into the spiritual aspects of DNA. Let's suspend our beliefs, if you will, for "suspension" is at the core function of an immortality code – the state of suspended cellular illumination.

Great News

At this time in humanities history, also referred to as the Great Awakening, we are now at a level of consciousness in which we are ready to receive the level of light necessary to activate more of our divine golden DNA, known throughout the cosmos as Diamond Human DNA.

The two strands of DNA we see now are activating into a greater expression and capable of 12, 24 and 144 strands, all multiples of 12. These are the codes of a fully activated divine being, living in a human body. Each strand is built upon 12 nucleotide-based chemicals. The fully active 12 strand DNA Template has 144 chromosomes, 12 chromosomes for each strand of DNA.

As this occurs, "we" become the form of humans we were designed to be. Truly divine beings. And every single one of us has this written within their DNA.

We study and we learn new lifestyle technologies and elixirs and we claim our limitlessness.

We become masters at communicating and commanding our cells, dialing in a new level of radiance, life force and true health. We choose our lifespan and, more importantly, we choose our quality of life along the way.

We train to carry more "light" within our bodies and we integrate ways to vibrationally uplevel our lifestyles and how we experience life on earth.

DNA is the interface with God. And when we perceive our DNA as a highly sensitive form of antennae that are communicating with our higher levels as well as our human levels, we understand spiritual epigenetics.

The Adam Kadman Body

In the Kabbalah, God's image of man is known and referred to as the Adam Kadman body. Leonardo DaVInci's drawing of the Vesuvian Man depicts a human in perfect proportions using sacred geometry, ratios and measurements such as the golden mean. The Adam Kadman is this and so much more. He is God in a body.

The Kabbalah also refers to a "primordial cell" within the Adam Kadman body. This cell contains all the fully activated DNA of the human potential – the 144 fractalization, which includes immortality. So we have a map we can trace back to re-activate our full potential.

In this way, immortality is a portal system. Just as one travels through thoughts and dimensions, one travels through the layers of our embodiment and physical bodies to the primordial cell. This is a state of consciousness where all is possible, especially the art of practicing suspended cellular illumination.

Consciousness is also another word for frequency. Everything has a code or a frequency and frequency changes everything.

This is where science and spirituality beautifully merge.

"Spirituality is just physics not yet understood."

–Nassim Haramein

Raising Our Frequency Protocols

The training to raise our frequency, or carry more light, is a series of vibrational stacking protocols. We are direct transmissions of frequency in every moment and we have agency over our frequency.

Of course, we start with an epigenetic lifestyle. How we eat, sleep and breathe. This book contains great detailed and researched material on these protocols. Here, let's look at them through a spiritual lens.

Eating

This is the manna of life. The infusion of life force. Pure, clean organic foods according to your genotype. Eating for results and higher performance instead of emotional needs. Blessing your food with divine intent. Sharing the intake of food with loved ones in uplifting environments.

Sleeping

This means getting at least 7.5 to 8 hours, time enough for the brain to detox itself. Understanding the dreamtime function, lucid dreaming and the ability to remember your dreams. Becoming deeply conscious and reverent of the regenerative function of sleep.

The Elegance of Breath

Ancient yogis mastered the breath and created different states of consciousness through different breath patterns, holds and rhythms. The yogi master, known as Desikachar, taught these practices for many years.

"In order to influence our prana we must be able to influence the mind. Our actions often disturb the mind, causing prana to exude from the body. Through daily pranayama (breathing) practice, we reverse this process, as a change in the breathing pattern influences the mind."

–TKV Desikachar

The ascended master Quan Yin, known as the Goddess of Compassion, is often depicted riding a dragon with a countenance of supreme calm and poise. To me, this is the perfect metaphor for mastering the breath and having the ability to choose your state of reaction and response to the world around us, no matter what the situation. Nothing could be more valuable at this time!

The science of breath covered in this book is amazing technology to learn how to control our CO_2 levels, keep our breath small, and activate optimal levels of serotonin and melatonin.

The field of plant medicine is gaining great popularity and phenomenal results for healing and awakening many individuals. Through the activation of DMT, one is able to see into and experience other realms where guidance, insight and divine "a-ha" alignments can happen.

Another way to activate one's DMT is through the practice of breathwork. This is gaining popularity and the results can be equivalent to the plant journey. I speak from personal experience on this and have incorporated breathwork into my weekly practices. I recommend working with a professional experienced breathwork guide, whose purpose is to create the perfect safe container for one to be free to experience massive dimensional journeys and expansion.

Meditation at its core function is to quiet the untamed thoughts and calm the mind. A simple meditation with breath practice is all that is needed with the sole purpose of relaxing into the infinite nature of this generous and magnanimous universe.

The simplest form of meditation is to count one's breath up to four, repeat and intend to feel the love of God.

Heart Coherence

Heart coherence is now accepted in all well-being practices as a beneficial state. It has been measured and proven initially by the organization known as Heart Math of California and has grown from there.

The heart contains seven chambers which, when working in resonance, create the heartbeat of God, or the "God Spark." This is the pulse of light and divinity produced by the frequency generator of the heart. The healing and resonance powers are enormous.

The deeper in meditation one can go into the resonance of heartspace, the bigger and brighter the field of energy unfolds into expansiveness consciousness.

A goal of meditation and good spiritual health is to live in heartspace as an ideal.

Sound Healing

Sound is frequency and vibration. Sound bowls, chanting, "om"-ing, and toning are some of the obvious ways of increasing our vibration through the art of sound. This is a large part of the future of healing and medicine.

Part of sound healing is the use of Divine Decrees which command the use of energy and light into higher purposes. They are light code, turned into frequency, morphed into words and then made manifest through the physical breath of the spoken word.

Vibrational stacking is just that, curating and surrounding oneself with the highest frequencies available in order to express and organize DNA into its newest, highest and most divine expression, on a moment to moment basis.

My Contribution

My work involves helping people find ways to live their highest version here on earth, and includes helping people find out exactly why they are here and what their higher destiny is.

"When you truly know why you are here on earth and what your divine assignments are, you don't age." –Dolores Canon

When one has clarity around their mission, they are able to focus and amplify their energy. It repurposes one's energy into divine alignment and out of confusion. This creates a field of coherence in one's entire life and we settle into a higher quality of life.

Humans spend enormous amounts of energy wondering why they are. This is a type of superpower when found and ignites us on a cellular level, the basis of spiritual epigenetics!

Beyond giving lifetime destiny readings and being a coach for visionary leaders, I love to help others incorporate the grand epigenetic lifestyle of body, mind, spirit and purpose. The whole cosmic enchilada!

Connect with me at: https://www.instagram.com/gisellekoy/

Giselle Koy *is a transformational couch who channels soul-fulfilling destinies for visionaries. She is known for helping people step into their full power on the world stage. Her gifts of divine clarity serve many people in positions of power. She speaks on "Turning Your Spiritual Gifts into Wealth" and has given keynote presentations on stages such as Paleofx, Cosmic Awakenings, Conscious Media Festival and others.*

As a certified Epigenetic Coach, Giselle speaks on the topic of Spiritual Epigenetics, an area where science and spirituality meet. She trains people to be more lit by combining spirituality with high performance training techniques, to look and feel younger and better than they ever have.

Giselle is the Founder of the Conscious Media Festival and Conscious Visionary Women, as well as a member of the Vanity Fair's Founder Fair. She is the host of the Giselle Koy Podcast, speaking with thought leaders about the New Human Emerging in this accelerated time of Earth's Ascension.

https://www.gisellekoy.com

SOLUTION

What you seek, is seeking you.

–Rumi

Welcome to the section where the wisdom, science, and knowledge all come together to share your longevity solution. While the information is universal, the path and how to precisely apply what answers will best work for you will be different for each person. This is why you are now invited in to take the longevity life assessment. It will offer clarity designed to meet you in this moment of your current health expression and desires to identify the immediate, short- and long-term opportunities available for you to live your most thriving longevity life.

CHAPTER THIRTY-TWO

The Longevity Life Assessment

Dr. Melissa Grill-Petersen

Figuring out your next best steps to increase longevity can be pretty confusing. From breath and gratitude practices to sirtuins, exosomes and peptides, it seems there are so many ingredients that need to be balanced to find the perfect recipe for you. To begin mapping out this journey, you must honestly assess two things – where you currently are and the desired outcomes you seek. That said, whether you are just getting started or you are ready to go to the next level of optimizing your system, your next steps will depend on your specific longevity stack.

The following longevity life assessment will allow you to immediately see the key areas of greatest personal potential for improvement.

Know that this is simply a suggested beginning point that will allow you to move along your optimization path. As you are ready for a more precise approach to achieve your desired outcomes and results by leveraging the latest age rejuvenation protocols, that is where myself and the contributors of this book come in over at the Longevity Experts Network. There you will find a complete directory of certified epigenetic coaches, doctors and clinicians of various specialties and degrees who work in a systems-based approach caring for the whole of you bringing a comprehensive plan that coordinates the outer world and inner health expression based on your genetic blueprints to express your fully energized, vital, longevity life.

Step One: Take the Longevity Life Assessment. As you have read throughout this book, if you desire to optimize your lifespan, healthspan and wellspan you MUST master the quality of the inputs coming into your system that inform the function and expression of your health. After the lifestyle assessment, there is an added guide that will determine if you could benefit from advanced therapies and clinical care to include strategies like hyperbaric oxygen, regenerative therapies, exosomes, hormones and peptides with our team of longevity experts.

Step Two: Review the Recommendations that are shown to be highly supportive based on your answers and areas of greatest need in supporting enhanced longevity.

Step Three: Make Your Plan. Determine your immediate, short- and long-term actions that you will take. Join our free group or work with one of our experts to personalize your path. To learn more, visit: www.CodesofLongevity.com

Let's Get Started

Begin your longevity assessment:

1. Undercover Your Longevity Potential

    a. Calculate your "longevity lifespan potential," which is the age of your oldest relative, minus your current age. This is your minimum lifespan potential.

    b. Next, ask yourself, *"How do you want to be living, feeling and experiencing this amazing longevity life of yours?"*

    c. It's essential to understand what you truly desire, why it matters, and how important it REALLY is for you so you can align with the actions that will support your desired outcome. Remember, if you have any emotional resistance, go back to Chapter One for a personal mind hack session.

2. Assess the Impact the Hallmarks of Aging Impact are Having on Your System

The nine hallmarks of aging are the physiological components that impact the rate at which your body ages. As discussed in various chapters throughout this book, each category has specific researched outcomes that are shown to positively improve the function.

Rate your subjective experience or symptoms as they pair with each hallmark. Based on your response you will be directed into a more targeted starting point on your path of precision longevity living.

Answer Y for yes, O for occasionally or N for no. Then total your score and divide it by the number of questions in each section. This will give you an idea out of the 3 sections where you should consider focusing the most first.

Hallmarks 1-4 focused on DNA expression and replication	Y- 2	O- 1	N- 0
Do you smoke?			
Do you consistently get six or fewer hours of sleep a night?			
Are you exposed to poor air quality or pollution frequently?			
Are you exposed to chemical toxins such as pesticides or herbicides on your food, in your lawn care, pest control or at work?			
Do you consume GMO foods that contain Glyphosates? (Main sources are foods made from or with corn, soy, wheat and rice.)			

Have you experienced emotional trauma or sustained psychological stress?			
Have you experienced mold or Lyme sickness?			
Do you experience regular allergies?			
Do you experience mood disorders with increased anxiousness or depression?			
Do you regularly drink unfiltered tap water that is fluoridated, in plastic bottles or flavored with artificial sweeteners?			
Total score (add it up and divide it by 10 to get your average)			

This section is key as it impacts all other biological functioning throughout the system.

Increased stress loads, be they chemical/environmental; mental/emotional; or physical can accelerate the rate of metabolic break-down and chaos in the system.

Immediate support in the literature is shown to include but not be limited to:

a. Lifestyle: breath, meditation, sleep restoration and re-sistance exercise training.

b. Nutrition: Anti-inflammatory, nutrient dense bioactive foods and hydration.

c. Wellbeing: Share your capacity for purpose by volun-teering, and connecting with others.

   d. Supplements: Genomic benefit can be gained from the use of Nicotinamide (precursor to NAD); Sulforaphane (found in broccoli and kale); Glutathione (absorption issues, must be in a lipid delivery system); Sirtuin support (Resveratrol and Pterostilbene); and essential methylation support: Folate, B6, B12, Betaine, Magnesium, and Zinc. Melatonin aids in DNA repair and replication.

   e. Advanced therapies: Peptide therapy (Epitalon & BPC-157 are foundational).

Hallmark 5-7 focused on cellular health, energy and vitality	Y-2	O-1	N-0
Do you experience low energy levels?			
Do you eat a diet high in carbohydrates, sugars and/or fried foods?			
Do you consume more than one alcoholic beverage a day?			
Are you diabetic or pre-diabetic?			
Do you consume GMO foods that contain Glyphosates? (Main sources are foods made from or with corn, soy, wheat and rice)			
Have you experienced emotional trauma or sustained psychological stress?			
Do you primarily eat convenience processed foods from a box, bag, can or drive thru?			

Do you have known hormonal imbalances or issues such as belly fat, difficulty losing weight, temperature dysregulation, mood swings, acne, thinning hair, sleep issues?			
Do you have a BMI over 30 or know yourself to be overweight by more than 20 pounds?			
Total score (add it up and divide it by 9 to get your average)			

This section impacts your body's energy and repair systems. Increased infection and compromised nutrition in quality, quantity, and absorption, as well as hormonal stressors, can all lead to a proinflammatory state. This can accelerate the rate of metabolic breakdown and chaos in the system, leading to an increase in senescent or "zombie" cells.

Immediate support in the literature is shown to include but not be limited to:

a. Lifestyle: Intermittent fasting, breathing techniques, meditation, sleep restoration, aerobic and resistance exercise training.

b. Nutrition: Glucose stabilization is key, moving towards a lower carb approach while increasing monounsaturated fats and lean proteins.

c. Wellbeing: Foster a sense of gratitude and happiness as it correlates with improved metabolic health.

d. Supplements:

　　i. B6 for blood sugar and cellular health support.

ii.   Metformin medication for AMPK activation and blood sugar control (Berberine is the natural supplement that acts in a very similar fashion to Metformin.)

iii.   Essential hormonal support of DHEA, Melatonin and Vitamin D3.

iv.   Advanced hormones to consider include thyroid and testosterone.

v.   Sirtuin support for optimal cellular energy: Resveratrol, Pterostilbene and or Nicotinamide (precursor to NAD).

vi.   Senescent cell removal with Fisetin, Quercetin and Curcumin, the most recognized and beneficial synolityics.

f.   Advanced therapies: Cold thermogenesis, hyperbaric oxygen, and biofeedback.

Hallmarks 7-9 focus on immune pathways and communication.	Y-2	O-1	N-0
Do you have consistent joint or body pain?			
Do you have an autoimmune condition?			
If you get a wound, does it heal slowly?			
Do you get sick easily?			
Do you have frequent infections?			

Do you feel tired often?			
Do you have skin rashes?			
Do you have digestive issues?			
Do you have a lot of stress in your life?			
Do you get less than ten minutes a day of outdoor sun exposure?			
Total score (add it up and divide it by 10 to get your average)			

Your immune health is your lifeline to enhanced vitality at any stage or age in life. To prompt natural stem cell production, thymus support and proper immune modulation for vibrant health, healing and regeneration, consider the following:

Immediate support in the literature is shown to include but not be limited to:

    a. Lifestyle:

          i.   Stress reduction through meditation to lower cortisol and boost sirtuin pathways.

          ii. Sleep optimization; leveraging daily morning and early evening sunlight exposure.

         iii. 20-30 minutes daily of varied exercise of mild to moderate intensity for natural stem cell stimulation. Rebounding on a trampoline is great for added detox and immune health.

b. Nutrition: Anti-inflammatory, nutrient dense bioactive foods and hydration.

c. Wellbeing: Random acts of kindness and generosity improve immune health. Foster greater happiness through gratitude noticing the daily moments of appreciation.

d. Supplements:

    i. Curcumin, ECGC, Glutathione (absorption issues, must be in a lipid delivery system).

    ii. Sirtuin support-Resveratrol and Pterostilbene.

    iii. Essential vitamin support: A, C, D and Zinc.

    iv. Essential hormonal immune support: Melatonin and DHEA.

e. Advanced therapies: Peptide therapy (Thymosin alpha and Thymosin Beta, GHK-Cu along with HGH) and Hormone therapy for adrenal and thymus support.

For the most complete understanding of your biological health optimization opportunities, you may want to consider a precision longevity work-up, including;

a. Blood work: Complete Blood Count (CBC); Comprehensive Metabolic Panel (CMP); Estradiol, Ferritin (iron storage); FSH (Follicle Stimulating Hormone); Hemoglobin A1c (HgbA1C), Homocysteine; hs-CRP, Insulin; LH (luteinizing hormone); Lipid Panel with Ratios; Lipoprotein Fractionation; Progesterone; Immunoassay; 25-Hydroxyvitamin D (D2, D3); T3 Reverse (RT3), LC/MS/MS; Thyroid panel (TSH, Free T3, and Free T4); Testosterone; Total and Free; Sex Hormone Binding Globulin and Thyroid Antibodies.

b. Genetic testing with epigenetic lifestyle reporting that covers: nutrition; sleep; stress, fitness/ performance; environmental detox; neurotransmitters; hormones; and supplementation. To order yours go to www.apeironzoh.com/codes

c. TruDiagnostic epigenetic age testing that uses methylation changes to the DNA readings for predictive outcomes in understanding biological versus chronological age. Since age is already the number one risk factor for all chronic diseases this makes sense, however, the test is exciting because it allows us to test how interventions are changing the risk of disease and lifespan immediately. This offers the ability to measure reverse aging that can occur when personalized changes are made and measured over time as paired with labs, genetics, and biometrics for the greatest level of precision health.

d. Dutch test for your brain neurotransmitters and hormonal health index.

e. Dexa or Inbody body composition assessment noting bone density, fat, muscle mass, BMI and phase angle.

f. qEEG brainwave assessment to ensure proper brainwave expression.

g. HRV – stress assessment to note the current state of your central nervous system.

h. Capnography as an advanced tool to assess CO_2/ O_2 levels in the tissues of the body.

i. Functional movement assessment noting muscular imbalances, gait and posture patterns to optimize for enhanced performance.

3. Assess Your Epigenetic Inputs

Take the next stage of this assessment to gain deeper insight and understanding into the immediate opportunities available in your daily life to optimize your longevity life.

Remember, epigenetics is the signal from "above the gene" or in other words, the inputs from the outworld, informing the inner world. *Science has shown it is a combination of biological, interpersonal and social factors combined that overall impact the expression of health and thriving in the human system.*

By taking a multifactorial or systems-based approach you will rapidly uplevel how you look, feel and live, and ensure that you continue on your path to a longer, optimized life!

Rate each interaction on a scale from 0-3 (0 is never, 1 is sometimes, 2 is often, 3 always)

Sleep				
I get 7-9 hours of quality sleep each night	0	1	2	3
I fall asleep and wake up around the same time daily	0	1	2	3
My sleep environment is optimized *(cool, quiet or white noise, dark, comfortable, etc.)*	0	1	2	3
I wake up rested and energized each day	0	1	2	3
I fall back to sleep easily if I wake up during the night	0	1	2	3
I do not eat or drink any grains, alcohol, sugar or caffeine within two hours or more of going to bed.	0	1	2	3

I minimize blue light exposure from my smartphone, computer, tablet or laptop at least 30-60 minutes prior to going to sleep.	0	1	2	3
My mouth is closed making minimal to no sounds during sleep	0	1	2	3
Total score (add it up and divide it by 8 to get your average)				

Sleep, across the literature, is THE essential key to optimized health and there is no hack around it. Consistently getting less than seven hours or more than nine hours takes a cumulative toll on the system, paired with adverse health outcomes including total mortality, cardiovascular disease, type 2 diabetes, hypertension, and respiratory disorders, obesity in both children and adults, and poor self-rated health.

The first step to improving sleep for system-wide health is to **make sleep a priority**. Next, focus on regulating your sleep schedule so that you're going to bed and waking up at the same time each day. The more light you get earlier in the day will support better sleep at night by programming your inner clock genes. Finally pay attention to what you do 2-3 hours prior to bed, including light exposure; foods (grains, alcohol, sugar, and caffeine); and optimizing your sleep environment (temperature, light, EM, and sound) for a path to deep, restorative sleep. Further exploration will include O2 levels throughout the night, brain wave activity and hormones.

Rate each interaction on a scale from 0-3 (0 is never, 1 is sometimes, 2 is often, 3 always)

Food				
I mainly eat fresh, local or organic foods	0	1	2	3
I eat nutrient dense, high quality ingredient meals	0	1	2	3
I minimize the amount of processed or fast foods I eat	0	1	2	3
I feel nourished & energized from the foods I eat	0	1	2	3
I seldom drink sugary or artificially flavored drinks	0	1	2	3
I seldom eat foods that upset my stomach	0	1	2	3
I seldom experience digestive issues	0	1	2	3
I take supplements for enhanced health support	0	1	2	3
I sit down to enjoy my meals without rushing sure to chew eat bite	0	1	2	3
I regularly practice time-restricted eating of at least 12 hours	0	1	2	3
I drink clean, filtered water throughout the day	0	1	2	3
If I microwave food, I do it in a glass container	0	1	2	3
I eat and drink out of glass or ceramic dishware	0	1	2	3
I have regular daily bowel movements	0	1	2	3
Total score (add it up and divide it by 14 to get your average)				

You are what you eat. Did you know that honey bees are genetically identical in a hive? Both the worker bees and the queen are genetically the same. The only difference is what they are fed. They all start out consuming "royal jelly" and within a few weeks the worker bees are switched over to a diet of pollen and nectar. What determines how they express are the signals informing their genetic code from the food they eat. We are just like bees. What we eat matters to how we express or repress thriving states of health.

Food is one of the most consistent and frequent input signals to the body. What, how, how much and when you eat all make a difference.

Notice the prompts in the questions. Any answer that scored a zero for "never" are the immediate opportunities to explore. For example, if you never sit down to enjoy your meals, this will impair digestion. You can aid your body's absorption by making a ritual out of mealtime, committing to slowing down, enjoying the food, and ensuring you chew 20 to 30 times. If you eat a lot of con- venience foods due to your schedule, you could make a com- mitment to replace some of those with meals you make at home and take with you.

Quality matters, especially at a genetic level. Do your best to reduce the frequency of consuming highly processed and pre-packaged foods, and choose organic over conventionally grown. Sustainably raised, wild-caught or free range are all higher quality with greater bioavailability to the system.

Rate each interaction on a scale from 0-3 (0 is never, 1 is sometimes, 2 is often, 3 always)

Movement				
I move for at least 20 minutes continuously daily	0	1	2	3
I walk and perform daily tasks pain free with comfort and ease	0	1	2	3
I perform resistance weight/training exercise at least two times per week	0	1	2	3
I vary the types of exercise and movements I do regularly	0	1	2	3
I get up after sitting to move every 45-60 minutes throughout my day	0	1	2	3
I have great balance and can stand on one leg for 60 seconds at a time	0	1	2	3
I have strong grip strength and can open things easily	0	1	2	3
I have excellent posture being sure to sit and stand tall	0	1	2	3
I seldom experience joint /body aches or pain	0	1	2	3
Total score (add it up and divide it by 9 to get your average)				

Across every hallmark of aging, exercise shows a positive impact on lifespan and healthspan while reducing all-cause mortality. Exercise targets every foundational longevity pathway in the body, so if you want to begin the reverse aging process, it's time to move.

Seek out play and patterns of movement that are enjoyable, varied and engaging for you.

Remember, the body thrives through diversity. Jot down at least seven different types of movement or activities you love to do or would do, such as: walking, gardening, yardwork, playing golf, dancing, resistance training, stretching, going for a bike ride with friends or family, et cetera.

From your list of ideas, make movement an essential part of your daily schedule. Twenty to thirty minutes a day is ideal. If you train too much or too hard with little recovery time in between workouts, you can actually speed up the aging process.

Using wearable technology like an Oura ring, Garmin watch or Whoop band will tell you how well your body is or is not recovering so you don't keep pushing the system into a state of distress. Remember, keep it varied, fun and engaging so each day you will help your body help you express your best.

Rate each interaction on a scale from 0-3 (0 is never, 1 is sometimes, 2 is often, 3 always)

Nature				
I breathe easily in and out through my nose for 8-12 breaths per minute	0	1	2	3
I get at least ten minutes of natural sunlight exposure daily	0	1	2	3
I get outside every day for at least 20 minutes	0	1	2	3

I have nature pictures or plants in my home, office or daily environment	0	1	2	3
I take time to connect and align with the pace of nature	0	1	2	3
Total score (add it up and divide it by 5 to get your average)				

Time in nature resets how our internal clock genes express. Tied into the circadian rhythm, our inner clocks impact our metabolic, hormonal and immune health, as well as our mental / emotional wellbeing.

When you are outside in the fresh air, proper breathing can be a simple and powerful way to increase your energy, focus and mood. Make a habit of going outside in the early morning light to practice box breathing – in through your nose for four counts, hold for four counts, out for four counts, and hold for four counts.

To take it to the next level, stand outside with your bare feet on the ground and, while sun gazing, do some focused box/nose breathing a minimum of ten minutes. If your work schedule is packed, take your meetings on the phone outside. You can also sit under a tree, go for a walk, or get some plants and bring nature inside your house.

Rate each interaction on a scale from 0-3 (0 is never, 1 is sometimes, 2 is often, 3 always)

Hormones/ Metabolics				
My body temperature is normal, seldomly running hot or cold	0	1	2	3

I have sustained energy levels daily	0	1	2	3
I have a close to ideal body weight and BMI	0	1	2	3
I have little to no abdominal "belly fat"	0	1	2	3
I have great mental clarity and focus	0	1	2	3
I have a full head of hair, healthy nails and eyebrows	0	1	2	3
I have good muscle mass	0	1	2	3
My mood is steady and my outlook on life is good	0	1	2	3
I am able to make clear decisions	0	1	2	3
I seldom, if ever, experience energy dips or cravings in the afternoon	0	1	2	3
Total score (add it up and divide it by 10 to get your average)				

The best place to begin optimizing your hormonal health is through stress reduction and resiliency.

Meditation, yoga, or tai chi are all proven practices that lower cortisol levels – a key driver of modern hormonal dysfunction.

No time? Box breathe. For a more optimized approach, it is ideal to do the suggested clinical workup to gain a complete picture of what is impacting the full expression of your health. This data can be ordered and reviewed with a precision longevity expert.

Rate each interaction on a scale from 0-3 (0 is never, 1 is sometimes, 2 is often, 3 always)

Stress				
I recover quickly from stress because I rest as needed	0	1	2	3
I practice stress reduction daily like meditation or breathwork	0	1	2	3
I practice some form of self-care daily	0	1	2	3
I am able to handle important situations or challenges easily in my life	0	1	2	3
I feel in control and/or on top of things in my life	0	1	2	3
I seldom ruminate or worry	0	1	2	3
If I get emotionally triggered, I center myself before responding	0	1	2	3
I track my resting pulse rate and it is often under 65	0	1	2	3
I track my Heart Rate Variability	0	1	2	3
Total score (add it up and divide it by 9 to get your average)				

Remember, stress is designed to serve a positive purpose in the body, but it must be paired with the ability to toggle back into a parasympathetic state of rest and recovery.

Stress is also different for everyone. Many of us don't even realize we're on "system overload" because abnormal has become our normal.

While too much of anything can be a stress to the system, here are some of the most common culprits: physical stressors, such as lack of sleep or injury; chemicals from tobacco, alcohol, drugs or medications; mental/emotional stress due to feelings of guilt, anger, worry, anxiety, depression or fear; and nutritional stressors brought on by allergies or sensitivities often triggered by GMOs or gut dysbiosis. You can also experience spiritual stress, for example, the loss of deeper meaning and connection.

To properly gauge your baseline to make an informed decision to the most optimal stress reduction strategies for you, track your biometrics. Whether you are taking your daily morning pulse or your HRV via more advanced wearable devices, you will begin to see and understand the state of health and resiliency of your system.

Tracking removes the guesswork so you can see the situation clearly and take informed action. You will see what is causing spikes and when you are not fully recovered; your body will also reveal what it wants and needs more or less in order to thrive.

As a beginning point, remember the three R's – Reduce, Reset, Rejuvenate. Reduce your exposure to the stress. Reset your system with proper rest and recovery. Rejuvenate by replenishing your system for new states of thriving.

Fundamentally, meditation is shown in the literature as *the* action to mitigate stress and positively impact more than 3,500 genes. Heartmath offers a fantastic app called Inner Balance that supports HRV coherence training. Improving vagal tone, as mentioned in Chapter Three, is your main toggle switch back into para-sympathetic states. In addition, advanced strategies such as biofeedback, neurofeedback and entrainment can all be beneficial to help your system become antifragile, resilient and robust!

Rate each interaction on a scale from 0-3 (0 is never, 1 is sometimes, 2 is often, 3 always)

Cognitive Performance				
I am able to focus for an hour or more at a time	0	1	2	3
I am able to recall long-term memories	0	1	2	3
I am able to recall short-term memories	0	1	2	3
I feel mentally clear and can make decisions easily	0	1	2	3
I learn and recall information easily	0	1	2	3
I am able to organize information easily	0	1	2	3
I remember words, names and numbers easily	0	1	2	3
I am aware of my stress and handle it well	0	1	2	3
I feel a sense of connection, ease and/or joy daily	0	1	2	3
Total score (add it up and divide it by 9 to get your average)				

Peak brain states drive mood, focus, clarity, memory and performance at any stage or age of life. Again, meditation is foundational, as it is shown to boost BDNF in the brain by over 280%.

Assuming you are sleeping, de-stressing and eating a nutrient-dense diet, you can next consider taking peptides (Cerebrolysin and biospecific hormones (cortisol support with DHEA and optimizing testosterone are paramount). Biofeedback through HRV coherence training, neurofeedback and PEMF aid in cognitive performance for both improved short- and long-term outcomes.

Rate each interaction on a scale from 0-3 (0 is never, 1 is sometimes, 2 is often, 3 always)

Environment				
I breathe in fresh, odorless, well ventilated air in my daily environment	0	1	2	3
The temperature in my environment is comfortable	0	1	2	3
The sound in my environment is non distracting or I wear noise protection	0	1	2	3
I easily focus on one task at a time	0	1	2	3
My work environment is comfortable	0	1	2	3
I minimize my exposure to blue light from electronic devices in the evening	0	1	2	3
I have colors, pictures and/or art work in my office and home environment that inspire me.	0	1	2	3
I use organic household cleaners and products	0	1	2	3
I use organic body products like lotions, makeup, and deodorant	0	1	2	3
I minimize my direct WIFI & EMF exposure	0	1	2	3
I have plants in my home and workspace	0	1	2	3

My environment is clean, organized, and clear from clutter	0	1	2	3
Total score (add it up and divide it by 12 to get your average)				

What do you notice from your answers? Do you have the opportunity to get more natural sunlight or to bring in plants and an air filter for better quality air? Your environment is critical, which is why we spend a lot of time in our 12 to 120 course sharing how to optimize this aspect of your life for enhanced states of thriving!

Just know that you can start with one step, one small change that can uplevel your health expression.

Rate each interaction on a scale from 0-3 (0 is never, 1 is sometimes, 2 is often, 3 always)

Wellbeing				
I have access to safe housing	0	1	2	3
I have access to healthcare	0	1	2	3
I have economic stability	0	1	2	3
I feel good about myself	0	1	2	3
I feel useful	0	1	2	3
I deal well with problems	0	1	2	3

I feel loved	0	1	2	3
I take time to laugh and play	0	1	2	3
I take responsibility for myself, health & happiness	0	1	2	3
I have a spiritual connection	0	1	2	3
I lead a purposeful and meaningful life	0	1	2	3
I have people in my life that we enjoy spending time together	0	1	2	3
I have a curious mind that stays open to new things	0	1	2	3
I feel optimistic about the future	0	1	2	3
Total score (add it up and divide it by 14 to get your average)				

Wellbeing is directly connected to your "wellspan." This is where your interpersonal experience expands into areas that are not as easily "measured" in the data. It's the magic evoked from things like purpose, love, appreciation, happiness and joy, community, collaboration, connection and consciousness. These aspects of self are the glue that tie a long, well-lived life together; and, when you share them with others, they spread across the planet and down to future generations to help everyone flourish.

So how to go about raising your score in this section?

Research shows that gratitude has immense physical, mental and emotional health benefits. A simple daily practice of noticing what went well, or the act of noticing what you are grateful for, will positively impact your health expression.

Each moment of each day there will be people, places, experiences and inputs to your system that you can't control, yet you can always be at choice how you perceive and respond to what is occurring around you.

Instead of letting the weight of that stress continue to impact your system, tip the scale in your favor by acknowledging the things (even the small ones) that *are* showing up for you and what truly is well in your body, health, relationships and life. When you look with open curiosity, ready to take notice of all that is good, the world will surprise and delight you in new and wonderful ways.

Understanding Your Epigenetic Assessment Results

Once you've completed the assessment you can start connecting the dots and begin making your action plan for enhanced health, vitality, and wellbeing. You want to build into this plan immediate, short-term and long-term steps that will keep you on your path.

First, let's celebrate YOU. Any item for which you scored a 3 or higher is optimized, so great job, no changes needed. Just keep doing what you are doing and build on that momentum.

Your overall score will consist of the average score of each section. The lower the number, the greater the need for attention and action.

Within each section, note your individual scores. You'll find that many actually reveal the exact action step to take. (For specific understanding or ideas, go back to the earlier chapters for more direction.) Note any "0" as immediate action sections requiring your greatest focus and attention, while "1"'s should be included in your short-term plan and "2"'s as part of your long-term plan.

- *Immediate points of action will require you to list out any and all "0" scores.* These are areas that require action now for rapid enhanced changes in your health expression.

- *Short-term action will include any "1" answers.* Of those, which are the top three you are WILLING to take action on over the next 30-45 days?

- *Your long-term strategy includes any "2" answers, along with remaining 1s and 0s.* Think of your 2's as items that you are doing pretty well with the majority of the time. Once you have made the key changes to any of your "0" or "1" then you can turn your long-term focus to optimize your experience with any of the items you selected as a 2 with the intention of moving them to a 3.

To live a long life, we must be committed for the long haul. Take this opportunity to look forward to what lies ahead. As you take inspired action from your assessment, know each choice is supporting you to more fully live your life, optimized.

Understand that this assessment does not require immediate attention on every item, rather, it is a framework to determine what really matters to YOU. Remember, you get to choose. No one is forcing you to take any action. Yet, IF you choose to act, based on what you have read and answered, now you know where to focus so you can experience the greatest gains the quickest.

You are now ready to start creating your action plan based on the data. Again, start with an immediate and short-term plan based on the areas where you currently have the opportunity to make changes or adjustments. The steps you can take are within your answers based on scores of "0" and "1."

Results Planning Example:

Category	Total Score	Immediate (0)	Short Term (1)	Long Term (2)
Sleep	1	*Go to bed and wake up around the same time daily.*	Improve sleep practices nightly *(cool room, reduce blue light, quiet, etc.)*	Get 7-9 hours of quality sleep each night.
Stress	2	Rest as needed so I can better recover quickly from stress	Begin a daily stress reduction practice of meditation or breathwork	Track my Heart Rate Variability
Nutrition	2	I eat too many processed or fast foods	minimize the amount of sugary diet drinks	Buy local and organic

You will see that sleep, stress and nutrition all need attention, but that could feel like a lot of changes at once. The idea is to create a plan that you WILL commit to acting on – in other words, one with small steps stacked on top of each other over time to create an amplified result.

If I had to choose one area over the other, I would choose sleep. Sleep is both the lowest score and impacts every aspect of biological health and function. It is also an area in which a few small yet specific actions can be taken so it's less likely to feel overwhelming.

Change occurs in small increments when actions are taken consistently over time.

If I tried to make myself change my food habits but I really wasn't fully ready, the likelihood of success and lasting change will be low.

Be willing to meet yourself where you are, but with a clear understanding of where you want to go, how you want to be living and WHY it's important to express enhanced health. The more you understand your why, the faster you will identify non-negotiables and find the inspiration you need to say YES to you.

If you were willing to do it all but had limited time, where would you start? You can see from the answers that part of the inability to manage stress is due to a lack of rest and recovery.

For example, if you're sleeping, you're healing, which means they're recovering and will be better able to respond and adapt during each day for enhanced health.

In the 12-to-120 course, we explain this process in depth to help you fully understand how you can design your precision plan.

For more resources, visit: www.CodesofLonevity.com

Now it's your turn: review your answers and turn the page to get a clear sense of how to put it all together in your personalized longevity stack.

CHAPTER THIRTY-THREE

Your Longevity Blueprint

Dr. Melissa Grill-Petersen

As you have probably come to realize in reading this book, while there is a general path to longevity maximizing it requires a personalized and precise approach aligned with one's unique genetic blueprint. Just as important, we must recognize that longevity encompasses not just lifespan, but healthspan and wellspan and therefore our approach must be a balance of biological strategies, lifestyle strategies, and interpersonal societal/social interactions. It is at this intersection that the magic occurs for you to express your best life, lived well.

Now you can begin to understand and appreciate that your body is a part of a whole, dynamic system constantly receiving and sending signals between the inner and outer world. Here you can zoom in and out to realize each piece connects to a larger whole that influences and aids in the design of your longevity blueprint for a thriving life.

To determine your path, you must assess where you are *at this moment*. This means being open and honest with yourself about how you are currently experiencing and expressing your health, vitality and performance. You then look at what you discovered when you took your longevity potential score and got inspired around how you WANT to be looking, feeling, and living. What, if any, opportunities came up?

Perhaps you added a few new adventures to your bucket list?

Maybe you decided life is meant to be enjoyed so why not start being more playful, loving and curious now?

You may have also realized upon taking your assessments that your body and life hold immediate keys to unlock your personal longevity potential. Actions that you can take over time to create your personal longevity stack.

Understanding the results of the assessment:

1. Review your lifespan drivers: These are in the three areas that create the nine hallmarks of aging. Which of the three requires your greatest support – DNA, cellular or immune?

2. Next, review your health and wellspan drivers. This information comes out of the nine epigenetic categories. Which requires your greatest support – Sleep, Nutrition, Movement, Nature, Hormones, Stress, Environment, Cognitive Performance or Wellbeing?

3. Finally, pair the hallmarks of lifespan with the epigenetics of health and wellspan to find your foundational longevity stack. Decide what you are WILLING to do and start there. For enhanced outcomes and accountability, visit www.CodesofLongevity.com for recommended providers and support.

Need Some Ideas to Get Started?

Here is an example of "ideal" longevity actions to set your blueprint day:

- Wake up rested after eight hours of quality sleep.

- Enjoy a sirtuin-friendly drink to promote metabolic health and age rejuvenation. Suggested is a cup of antioxidant rich matcha or green tea, or hot water with fresh turmeric, ginger and lemon. Let them be free from any sweeteners to maintain a fasted state, aiming for at least 12-14 hours since the last meal the night before.

- Maintaining optimal O2/CO2 and NO3 levels throughout the day by breathing at 8-12 breaths per minute. Keep the breath smooth, soft and gentle, in and out through the nose, not the mouth.

- Take ten minutes each morning to enjoy natural, early morning sunlight and "earthing" by standing bare feet on the ground to attune your body clocks and natural rhythm to the cycles of the earth.

- While earthing outside, amplify this expression with a 10- to 20-minute walking/movement session and verbalize what you are grateful for, or appreciative of. This will allow you to tune in, notice all that is good and happening for you in your life, and align your day with eustress.

- Hydrate throughout your day. Ideal recommendations are to take your body weight (in pounds) and divide that number by half. Drink that amount (in ounces) of clean pure filtered water. For example, if you weigh 120 pounds you should be drinking 60 ounces.

- After coming back from your morning nature walk of gratitude, perform dry brushing to stimulate lymphatic drainage of toxins or waste while aiding in skin exfoliation. Follow this up with shower, starting off at a cold temperature for 1-5 minutes, then a normal temperature. This enhances cognitive function, stimulates brown fat and regulates cortisol.

- Practice time-restricted eating. Enjoy a nourishing first meal of healthy fats, complex carbohydrates and protein, ideally 12-14 hours after your last meal of the previous evening.

This will stabilize blood sugar and keep you nourished and energized throughout your day for optimal brain and body health.

- Ensure that your work environment is ergonomically optimized for excellent posture. Also, practice time-blocking your day, allowing for movement breaks every 45-60 minutes, with 5- to 15-minute breaks for maximum efficiency and flow.

- Ensure that your daily environment includes exposure to clean air, reduced noise, nature in the form of art or plants and pleasant colors, and photos and sounds that inspire you and keep you in the flow.

- Eat high-quality, nutrient-dense meals containing 20-30 grams of protein (because protein is the currency of longevity), along with monounsaturated fats and complex fibrous carbohydrates such as greens and colorful veggies, which will meet your nutrient needs and give you energy throughout the day.

- Set healthy boundaries and ensure that you end your work day with plenty of time to enjoy all of the people, places and things that matter to you in life.

- Love what you do and do what you love. Live a life of purpose by honoring that nudge from within to experience things that inspire, engage and ignite you. Find a way to share this or support another source in your purpose-filled joy.

- Align with the rhythms of nature and honor your evening as a time to slow down by reducing technology and blue lights from devices. Turn off extra distractions like tv, games or social media that would otherwise keep your system amplified and activated so you can prepare for deep, restorative sleep.

- When worry strikes, acknowledge it, understanding that it's inviting you into a new state of awareness. Practice gratitude or the "What Went Well" exercise each night to notice any concerns or worries, then focus on at least 2-3 additional things that you are grateful for.

- Make quality sleep a non-negotiable. Value it as one of the essential components to a long thriving life. Getting 7-9 hours is the key to optimized metabolic health and ensures that you will be ready and energized for the day ahead.

Use wearable technology like the Oura ring, Garmin, Fitbit or Whoop, which will help you develop greater "interoception" – or the practice of self-awareness paired with active biofeedback from your body. This will give you massive understanding and insight into how your body IS responding to the inputs from your daily life. Don't guess, because if you are just getting started what you think is "normal" may often be abnormal.

That said, this information won't be of much value unless you use it. For example, if you are not fully recovered from yesterday, it is even more important to ensure that you don't keep pushing your system today. Remember, stress is good when there is recovery, so do everything you can to help your system to adapt, evolve and thrive.

Remember, longevity IS the long game – an adventure to be enjoyed. Though there are many moving parts, realizing the full benefits is easier than you think. Take cues from nature's rhythm and flow. Attune yourself, notice the goodness that is showing up for you, look ahead, plan ahead, and realize that there is so much more thriving to be experienced.

Still want more?

- Cycle your food to match the seasons, bringing color, textures and diversity. Honor the natural elements like dark and light, heat and cold. Be flexible like a willow tree blowing in the wind and resilient like grass growing through the concrete always finding a way to meet the light.

- Volunteer and extend support to others, remembering that connection and belonging are fundamental human needs.

- Challenge yourself by taking on a new skill, role, travel, workout, or environment, remembering that a challenge is a stress and the gain comes once you allow your system to rest for recovery into growth.

- Reduce, Replace, Replenish, Rest and Rejuvenate. It's a constant process, a little every day adds up like compounding interest producing a "net-net" exponential positive gain!

- Say yes more often to what inspires, excites and delights you while saying no thank you to more obligations that no longer serve you.

- Ask new questions, open yourself to learning. Learning is a key to longevity.

- Be curious; the world will surprise and delight you if you are curious to see what more is possible.

- Lengthen time, always looking forward to more that is to come. Life is unfolding for you!

As you begin to set in motion the foundational practices listed here and are ready to become more precise, visit all of the authors and me at www.codesoflongevity.com to gain additional resources to support you along the way.

And now my friend, I invite you to take inspired action, to set your vision into motion. If you ever feel overloaded, know that there are incredible clinicians around the globe (many offering virtual services) so you never have to go it alone. Your potential IS limitless, and you now hold the key to unlock your codes to longevity.

In Our Limitless Expression,

Dr. Melissa Petersen & the entire Codes of Longevity Authors Team

NEXT STEPS

For a full list of references and resources for this book, please visit:

www.CodesofLongevity.com

To access the Path to 120 digital course taught by Dr. Melissa sharing a self-guided path into applying the codes of longevity for enhanced vitality and wellbeing, visit:

www.CodesofLongevity.com

To begin your precision longevity adventure, visit:

www.LongevityLifeHub.com/Precision

For ongoing resources, podcasts, classes and content shared out by our experts, visit:

www.LongevityLifeHub.com

ABOUT THE AUTHOR

Dr. Melissa Grill-Petersen is a sought-out expert in thriving! An author, speaker and visionary leader in epigenetics and precision longevity, she connects the dots for experts and enthusiasts alike. Her work is the bridge between science and soul revealing the path of pure possibilities for those that are ready to unlock their code and harness their limitless potential to flourish and thrive while looking, feeling and living their life optimized.

She is the founder of Impact Inc, home to Longevity Life Hub & Longevity Experts Networks and holds the position as the Chief Limitless Officer and Director of Apeiron Academy of Epigenetics training coaches around the globe.

Her clinical training and background include: a Licensed Doctor of Chiropractic & Epigenetic Human Performance Success Coach, with a Board Certification in Holistic Health and a Masters in Wellness Leadership and Performance. Pair this with her past fitness and television career in the world of professional wrestling and you get a powerhouse that is on a mission to uplift, inspire and ignite people around the globe to express their full potential.

She is a seer of what is possible, holds the vision, and is paving the way for enhanced states of health, wellbeing and human flourishing that will positively impact the world for generations to come.

For more information visit:

www.DocMelissa.com
www.LongevityLifeHub.com
www.instagram.com/drmelissagp

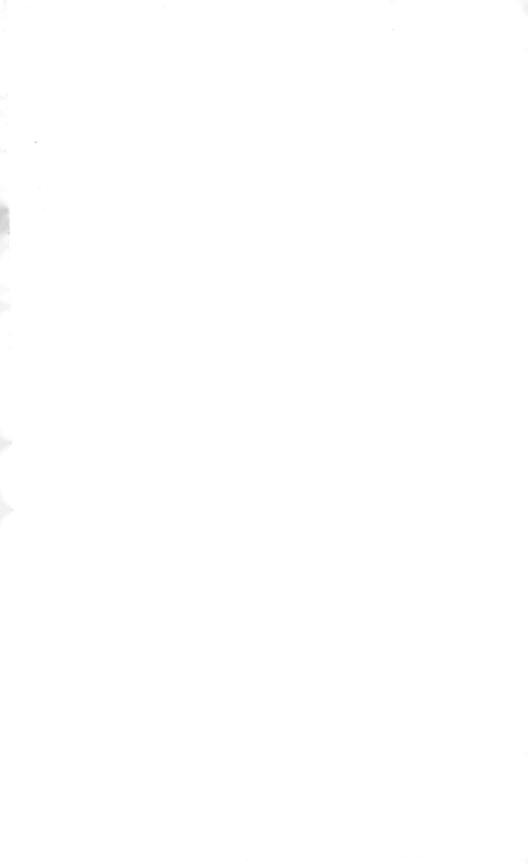

Made in the USA
Columbia, SC
15 August 2024

40483993R00180